Where's Mum?
Stories of Love, Loss And Menopause

Dr. Michael D. Meyer

This book of short stories is intended for informational and educational purposes only. It is not a substitute for professional medical advice, diagnosis, or treatment. The experiences, opinions, and insights shared herein reflect personal stories and research at the time of writing and should not be interpreted as medical guidance or as a comprehensive account of all aspects of menopause. Readers are advised to consult a qualified medical/healthcare professional or specialist before making any changes to their health care, diet, lifestyle, medication, or treatment plans. Neither the author nor the publisher assumes any liability or responsibility for any loss, injury, or damage incurred as a result of the use or misuse of the information contained in this book.

The publisher and author have made every effort to ensure that the information in this book is accurate and up-to-date at the time of publication. However, medical knowledge and understanding of menopause continue to evolve, and readers are encouraged to seek current, evidence-based information from trusted medical sources. All names, identifying details, and presentation of individuals have been changed or anonymised where appropriate to protect privacy. Any resemblance to actual persons, living or dead, is purely coincidental.

ISBN: 978-1-0685633-7-9 Printed in the European Union.

*Book Hub Publishing uses paper sourced only from sustainable forestry. Viva la forests!

We are committed to diversity, inclusion and equality.

Cover design and text layout by Niall MacGiolla Bhuí, ShadowScript Wordsmiths.

CONTENTS

Table of Contents

Introduction

The journey that led to this book was one of extensive research, hours of communication with powerful women, shocking discoveries, and self-healing. My healthcare education as a doctor of chiropractic meant that the information I studied was easy to comprehend (at least on a surface level), but by and large, it was totally new to me. I had no formal education about the menopause in graduate school, as is the case for most types of doctors in various health and medical fields. That is shocking, unacceptable and needs to change. I understand that it is unusual and possibly foolish for a man to write about this topic, as it is strictly a process that only a woman undergoes; however, while conducting my research, it became evident that loved ones are also affected to varying degrees. Not physically affected, of course, but affected nonetheless.

The short stories in this book are fictional with a hint of fact based on social media posts. My hope is that couples find a small nugget of familiar truth in a story that makes them feel less isolated on their individual and collective journeys. Writing this book genuinely helped save our marriage, and I desire to provide a platform of discussion to potentially do the same for others.

The first story encapsulates a narrative where a very young son tries to help his mum with his nan's help and is inspired to become a doctor in the future. This is followed by a story about a couple who try to work things out during a difficult period, which I revisit later. The third story is based on a radical change of personality and circumstance, and I revisit it later as well. The next one is set in rural Ireland and is tragic, as is the following story. Alternative options are explored in the following story, where a doctor must rely on options that pharmaceutical companies don't offer. Tragedy (yet again!) is the inspiration for the next one. I revisit two earlier stories next, and end my input with the longest story, which presents two different outcomes for the couples involved. The final story is a heartfelt contribution from project collaborator Catherine, who sheds light on the all-to-familiar haze of brain fog that so many women quietly endure.

I'm not an expert on the themes in this book. Rather, I see myself as a messenger who breaks the shrouded bubble of silence around menopause to encourage wider and deeper discussion. This book has the potential to promote resolution for many people if they approach it with open hearts and minds. The stories are purposely written in a format of *problem, resistance, breakthrough* and finally, *resolution*. The sentence structure is simplistic, and the dialogue is straightforward. It is meant to be an easy read where people can choose which chapter order they want to read. This book isn't intended to be a literary masterpiece, but rather a fictional blueprint to navigate the challenging conversations that need to happen for couples to emerge on the other side of the menopause.

Foreword

This is one of the bravest books in which I've ever taken part, written by one of the most tenacious individuals I've ever known. Michael first came to me as a very low and fractured human. His diet, lifestyle and very existence were on a self-saboteur's path to destruction. He was in need of a complete reset in his life, his 'mid-life' crisis being one of the mind, body and spirit, just as many women often endure when transitioning from the nurturing energy of the mother to the wisdom and strength of the crone during peri-menopause and the years which follow. I knew right from the start that he had the potential to emerge from his chrysalis of pain with a body of work which could be truly original and unique, enhancing the lives of all who would read it.

Michael has immersed himself, heart and soul, into this project in order to assist anyone who wishes to understand the menopause phase of the human life and how deeply it affects, not only the experiencer, but everyone around her. Not too many men would risk the wrath and ridicule of such an undertaking, but Michael has taken his own invaluable experiences, interviewed countless patients and friends, creating a book that I am certain will have people weeping, laughing, smiling and most importantly, healing.

Dr. Mary Helen Hensley
Book Hub Publishing, Head of Diversity, Inclusion and Equality,
Best-selling Author, Chiropractor, Healer
www.maryhelenhensley.com

WHERE'S MUM?

The change in Ben's Mum, Ann, was gradual. So gradual, in fact, that Ben didn't notice until she missed a cup final match shortly after his twelfth birthday. As he looked back years later, Ben could point out apparent changes in Ann's behaviour, but missing that match was unbelievable. He and his older brother, MJ, were the family's focal points as they grew up. Ben knew they were fortunate kids. They never lacked for anything and were somewhat spoiled as they took several holidays each year. Many times, his Nana, Una, on his Mum's side, would go along. These were the best because they got along well and did everything together.

Football was almost a religion to Ben and Ann. The boys had training or matches nearly every evening. Ann was a massive fan. Not only was she a fan, but she also played at an elite level in college. Ann had a goals record that stood for over ten years at university, and Ben was proud that his Mum wasn't just a cheerleader but also very knowledgeable about the game. None of his friends had a Mum like her. She was the hero he aimed to be. His dad, Stephen, usually went to the pub every evening after working long hours during the day. He never really played football like she did. Football was all Ben cared about.

Ben, now a grown man with a wife going through the menopause, can look back and clearly see the massive changes that gradually occurred in Ann. Nobody ever talked about that subject back then. People are only now starting to mention it in certain circles, but it's definitely not discussed enough. Ann was the rock of the family, while Stephen was the breadwinner. He made a very comfortable living as a second-generation electrician. The family unit was tight, happy, and active. The craic was always massive; it was rare to have any disharmony in the house.

Back in the early years, Ann coached Ben as an under-8s player. He loved that she was there for every training session. She would drive two or three of his friends' home after each session, and they would chat about absolutely anything and everything related to the game. When Ben moved up to the under-9s, he expected Ann to continue coaching. She didn't.

"Mum, why aren't you coaching me this year?" Ben asked Ann. "Ben, love, I need a break for a season," she replied. She felt a bit overwhelmed with everything that needed to be done around the house. She often felt tired, and didn't want to consider coaching a chore. "I'm sure I'll be back soon," she wasn't.

During that first-year break, Ben remembered that Ann began to spend much more time alone. Ann would take long walks and eventually started running on mountain trails, keeping her gone for long periods of the day. She always went alone. Ann explained that she needed the space to clear her head.

Ben remembered the joking banter his parents shared seemed to have all but completely disappeared during this period as well. There were some days when things were exactly like the past. Ann would drive him and MJ to training and stay for the entire session. The lads scrambled to get a lift home with her when the session ended. On those evenings, his parents might have a bottle or two of wine and snuggle on the couch to watch the telly. They teased each other and chatted cheerfully. Those days were getting fewer and fewer. Ben recalled that the banter sometimes sparked arguments or harsh words between his parents on different days. He also noted that Una didn't come around very often anymore, and when she did, many times, there would be loud talking, almost shouting, coming from the kitchen, which he didn't like at all.

They continued to take a couple of holidays a year as a family, but they were always shorter than they used to be. When Una went along, it wasn't the same. Ann and Una would barely talk; if they did, it was because they had to. They may have had to chat in a restaurant or at the airport, but otherwise, they hardly even looked at each other. The holidays they took without Una weren't any better. Ann began *exploring* on her own for many hours of the day, so the family would continue trying to have a holiday without her. Ann never returned to coaching. She rarely attended a training session; if she did, Ann would sit in the car and wait. She would always bring the two dogs, so there was no room for his friends to get a lift. Ben didn't mind because the trip home wasn't fun anymore. It was quiet. There was no advice, praise, or criticism, only silence. He wondered what he'd done to make his Mum not like him anymore. The cuddles, the fist bumps and the mussing of Ben's hair all vanished. Ben couldn't explain it to himself. He felt sad and mad because this was the new normal, and he couldn't figure out what he was doing to cause this.

The cup final was on a Saturday, and Ben had been aiming for that date the entire season. There was no guarantee they would be triumphant, but that was his goal from the first training session of the season. The day had finally arrived, but Ann wasn't home when he woke. Ben assumed that she must've gone for an early morning run. He would see her at the final later. Una arrived to drive them to the match. Stephen, MJ and Ben climbed into her car as she cranked up the tunes to get Ben psyched.

During the warm-up, Ben kept looking at the entrance gate whenever a car pulled into the car park, but none was Ann's. At kick-off, Ben decided to focus on the match and forget about everything else, as this match was an entire season in the making. Ben played about as well as a lad that age can, and his team was all playing some of the best football they'd ever played. The match was level 1-1 going into the final minute of injury time. Ben made a run and received a perfect pass from the corner. He jumped higher than he thought possible and smashed the ball into the corner of the goal with a powerful header. That was the last action of the match, as the referee blew the final whistle when the goalkeeper kicked the ball out. He tried to look for his family but was tackled to the ground by his centre-back for the goal celebration.

Ben's teammates mobbed him. He was at the bottom of a pile of the happiest young lads alive at that moment in time. It was a dream come true. The team got up and ran around the pitch like the professionals did at a Champions League Final, even though there weren't many people. Ben desperately looked for Ann as he circled the pitch. The players then climbed the bleacher steps to collect the cup. Ben, the captain, was handed the cup.

When he finished giving the customary acceptance speech, Ben locked eyes with Una and Stephen, then unmistakably mouthed the words. 'Where's Mum?'
Ben saw them both share a sideways glance, then look down at their feet. They apparently didn't know where Ann was either. It was the biggest day of his young life, and the person who had taught him how to do what he had done was

nowhere to be seen. Ben panicked. Ann went out early, so it was most likely into the mountains, and now he was worried that something tragic had happened. Ben dashed over to them and told them what he was thinking. They had been thinking something similar. Everyone figured she would turn up at some point during the match.

Ann's car was in the driveway when they pulled in, and they were all relieved. However, Ben immediately ran into the house to ensure she was okay. Ann was sitting at the kitchen table in her running clothes, drinking a cup of tea. He noticed that she looked fresh, as if she hadn't even run. He was now getting angry.

"Mum, what's wrong? Where were you? We won, and I scored the winning goal. I was so worried something bad happened to you," Ben blurted at machine gun pace.

"Congratulations," Ann said as she began to sob. She shook her head back and forth and placed her head in her hands and meekly tried to explain. "I went to the woods car park and sat there for a few hours. I didn't feel like running and thought I'd bring bad luck to you at the match. I knew you'd win if I didn't go, and I was right," Ann continued as the tears streamed. She then stood and wandered towards the lounge room in a daze.

Ben couldn't believe what he was hearing. What she said made no rational sense at all. Ann had been saying and doing things that were way out of character for her, and this was another unusual idea with no basis in reality. Ann was beginning to live by a strange set of rules that only she understood. Anger and confusion flooded him, and Ben had no idea what to say as she ambled slowly away. He wanted to tell her about the match, but she seemed so disinterested that he just let her go.

Ben had a shower and couldn't get his mind off what his Mum had said. He was going to have to ask a few serious questions. He wasn't looking forward to it, but it needed to be done. Ben dried himself off, dressed in a tracksuit and turned off the bathroom light. Una was sitting where Ann had been when he entered the kitchen. Ann was nowhere to be seen, and Una motioned for him to sit down.

"Ben, darling, you played every bit as well as your Mum ever did today, and I'm so proud of you. Your Mum is very proud too, even if she hasn't said it. She hasn't been herself for some time now, and I know why. Have a seat there; I have a story for you," Una said.

Una offered him a glass of water, orange juice, and a banana. She said it was for hydration, energy, and recovery. Una knew a lot about things like this. Ann learned from this wise woman, and now Ben was learning from her as well. Una took a deep breath and told Ben a story about herself when she was Ann's age in a manner that a twelve-year-old boy could understand. He couldn't believe what he was hearing. This single conversation changed the course of his entire life.

"I went through what your Mum's going through. All women go through it," she explained. "We called it *the change.* It's called the menopause. It happens to all women at a certain time in life. When I was Ann's age, there wasn't anything really to help, so I was given tablets to help me relax." Una continued, "They didn't work and made me feel like I was going crazy.

"Is Mum on tablets that make her the way she is?" Ben asked.

"I wouldn't be surprised; very few doctors know how to treat the menopause, but some do," Una explained.

Ben understood that certain things now made sense if his Mum was on tablets.
"I found a special doctor who can help Ann, but I can't convince her to go. She doesn't think anything is wrong, and I can't talk to her about it. She gets mad at me if I even mention it," Una said. "Maybe you give it a go. You two have a very special bond. Ann might listen to you, Ben," Una finished.
"I'll try, Nan; I just want my Mum back like she was when she was my coach," Ben said.

Ben immediately decided he couldn't be angry with his Mum any longer. He was on a mission to help her. After all, she was the reason he was a cup winner. Ben had to try to do something, anything.

Ben went into Ann's bedside locker when she was out. He found the tablets that Una had talked about. The container said Valium. Una had said they could make a person do unusual things. He immediately felt better inside himself because he could now sort of understand that it was the tablets making his Mum strange, and it didn't have anything to do with him. But now, the hard part. How will he convince his Mum to stop the tablets and see the special doctor that Una had found? He decided to simply be direct and bring it up whenever they were alone at the first chance. That's how a good football coach would handle this, and she was one of the best.

Ann came home at about half eight in the evening and seemed to walk like a zombie into the loo. Ben heard the shower and decided it was time to try talking to her when she got out. He went to his bedroom mirror to look at himself while he did his speech as the shower ran. Ben was more nervous than before the kick-off at the cup final, as he knew this meant so much more in life. The shower turned off, and Ann came out, draped in two towels as usual, one around her body, the other on her head. She went to her bedroom to dry off and blow-dry her hair. Ben practised one more time in the mirror while the hair dryer was going. The blow dryer stopped, and he knew that now was the time. Ben was petrified.

Ben knocked on the door and cautiously entered. Ann was lying on the bed with freshly blow-dried hair and a towel covering herself. The room smelled like heated shampoo and conditioner. This was one of Ben's favourite smells in the world. She used to come to tuck him in smelling like this, and he really missed that. Ben reminded himself he was there on a mission, so he came straight out and said it.

Ben had prepared what he was going to say, but instead of his speech, he began to blurt out one point after another in rapid succession while inhaling in short breaths. "Mum, I had a chat with Nana. The tablets you're taking are making you *not, Mum.* Everyone is worried about you. Nana said she knows of a special doctor who can help. She said this doctor knows of new things your doctor doesn't. Nana said I scored a brilliant goal, and you'd be sad you missed it if you saw it. I really, really miss you, Mum," Ben finished, then collapsed in a heap on her bed and began to cry and cry and cry.

Ann bent over, collected Ben into her arms, and then shared the cry. They sobbed for ages, and both felt better when they finished. They even giggled a little at the end.

Ann took Ben's head into her hands, looked deeply into his eyes, and shockingly said, "You and Nana are right. I need to do something different, and I need to trust Mum." When Ben woke, Una was at the kitchen table with Ann, having a cup of tea. There weren't any loud words. Instead, it was a calm and serious chat. He recognised that he shouldn't be there, so he took his overnight oats and went to the lounge room. Ben cheered like hell inside because Una could help get his Mum back, and he was hopeful for the first time in ages. Ben thought a quick trip to the special doctor to get new tablets would be all that was necessary.

Ann was no better in Ben's eyes three months after the special doctor visit. She said she was beginning to feel a bit better, but she still stayed alone, and he could tell any hugging from her felt forced. Ben needed to chat with Una as soon as he could. Thankfully, she was coming over for Sunday dinner. He was getting worried that it wasn't working.

When dinner was finished, Ben helped clear the table so he could hang around the kitchen and maybe get Una alone. It worked. Ann said she was tired and was going to lie down for a while. Stephen was off to the pub, and MJ only ever came into the kitchen to eat, so he was long gone. Una knew what was happening in Ben's head, so they sat at the kitchen table. She reached across and grabbed his youthful hands in her wrinkled ones full of love. She said, "Patience, Benjamin." He nodded and started to say something, but Una squeezed his hands and repeated, "Patience."

Ann had another visit to the special doctor a few months later, and a few months after that, Ben was pretty sure Ann was getting better. A further few months, he was certain she was returning to herself. Ann began to hang around the family in the evenings, and Ben could snuggle up next to her on the couch again, watching football matches. Ann began going shopping with Una again and occasionally attending their matches. She still didn't seem to get along with Stephen, but Ben hoped that would change. 'Patience,' he remembered as Stephen left for the pub.

They decided on Spain as the first family holiday in two years. Ann and Una were as close as ever, and he felt he had his Mum back. She was different from the football-obsessed version. Ann was calmer and less intense about things. Ben thought he wanted his old Mum back, but he loved this version even better somehow. Ben remembered Una saying that his Mum might be different when they figure out what works best for her. That had always worried him as Ben simply couldn't imagine a better version of his Mum, but he finally understood what she was saying. This version was just perfect, in his opinion.

Day three of the Spanish holiday was a massive turning point for the family. Ben was sure he'd heard intense, *quiet arguing* from his parents' room overnight. At breakfast, Stephen and Ann didn't so much as glance at each other. When they had finished eating, Ann and Una shared eye contact. They both stood up simultaneously and walked away from the table. Ben's mind raced as he knew something massive was happening. Stephen folded his arms across his big beer belly, leaned back in his chair, looked at Ben and his brother, and sighed.

Stephen cleared his throat and began, "Ben, MJ, I'm sure you know how difficult the past two years have been. I spent most evenings away from the house, waiting for your mother to go to bed, and I got up early to leave before she woke, so we didn't get into any arguments. Over that time, we have grown apart. Too far apart to find our way back to each other. I'm flying home this afternoon and moving out of the house before you all go home four days from now," he explained.

Ben was shocked to the core. He looked at MJ, who seemed much less shocked. Stephen and MJ shared a glance that implied MJ already knew what Stephen was going to say. Ben was a Mummy's boy, and MJ was far closer to Stephen, so even though it surprised him that his brother knew, it made sense that his dad would have had to be talking to someone. He now understood it was his brother. Ben was speechless.

The next big surprise came the following week when MJ and Ann had a loud screaming row in the kitchen just after training. It had been boiling since Stephen left Spain early.

"You don't have a fuckin clue how I feel about you and Da splitting. You forced him out by being a bitch," MJ roared.

A stunned Ann screamed, "You have no right to speak to me like that. You've no idea what hell I've been going through the past couple of years. Yer Da likes the drink more than he likes me. I didn't ask him to leave; it was his idea, but I'm happy he's gone."

It got louder and louder, and finally, MJ threw his kit bag into the corner and stormed out of the kitchen.

"I'm outta here!!! I'm moving in with Da," MJ roared at the top of his lungs.

Ben had no idea where to look as MJ brushed past him on the way to his room. Ann was in tears, so Ben rushed to her and wrapped his arms around her. MJ spent the afternoon packing his things, and Stephen collected him just before dinner. Una came over for the meal to comfort Ann, then spent the night in the now-empty bedroom. Una stayed over many times over the next few weeks, chatting with Ann late into the night. Ben loved having her there.

Una put her house for sale and moved in permanently with Ann and Ben. It was a crazy game of shifting people, places, and things, and Ben felt anxious that nothing would settle and that this chaos would be his life from now on.

However, things calmed down, and home life was pretty good after a few months. Ann and Una were more like sisters or friends, and Ben was flying in football. He was looking forward to the cup final again, as they were going for three in a row that year. Ann was going to be there for sure. He saw Stephen and MJ almost every day before or after training, and MJ was apprenticing to be a third-generation electrician. They were happy living together. Ben couldn't have imagined a scenario like this in his wildest dreams, and if he could've, he certainly never believed everyone involved would be mostly happy. Stephen seemed lonely and refused to go down the divorce path because couples just didn't do that. This part made Ben sad.

They won the treble and became the first team to win three consecutive titles in that division. The party in the local pub after the match was incredible. It was at that celebration that Ben met a certain girl whom he now calls his wife. She is a beautiful woman who is madly passionate about football, and she played at the same college his Mum did all those years ago.

Ben's wife, Jill, is now forty-two years old. The past year has been physically challenging for her. "I'm too young to be in perimenopause," she said to Ben after he suggested HRT.

"Jill, my love, I know what I'm talking about. Trust me," Ben gently replied, wrapping his arms around her.

Ben's chat with Una about his Mum all those years ago led him into medical training. He completed his degree in Ireland and then spent a year in the UK undergoing intensive training on the menopause. He is the leading specialist in the area and one of the very few males with this unique training in Ireland.

Jill hated to admit it, but she knew deep inside he was right. She returned the hug and quietly replied, “What’s next, Benjamin?”

Ben looked her in the eyes and said, “Explore available options and be patient.”

MARRIAGE COUNSELLING

JP had calmly entered the kitchen a few hours earlier, cleared his throat, and made deep eye contact with Maggie. He quietly stated, “I've been thinking about our relationship for well over a year. Anytime I’ve tried to talk to you, you’ve shut me down.”

“Don’t be daft. What on earth are you talking about?” Maggie responded as she glanced up from her computer. She was watching RTE News and obsessed with social media, as always, and didn’t fully register what he was saying.

“If you have a long, hard think about how you’ve treated me and everyone close to you the past couple of years, I’m sure you’ll figure out what I mean,” JP quietly replied. “I’m sorry it's come to this, but I can’t see any other way. I understand you are going through a type of living hell on some days, and I hate to see you like that.”

“What do you mean?” Maggie interrupted in an aggressive but shaky voice before JP had finished talking. JP continued, “I’m too young not to have pleasant conversations with a companion in the future.” “I don’t have the slightest idea what you’re on about,” she countered. “You do,” he finished. He handed Maggie an envelope and picked up his small suitcase. He turned and walked slowly out of the kitchen. Maggie heard the front door quietly close before opening the large manila envelope and was shocked to the core by its contents.

The divorce papers were spread out before her on the table, and her cup of tea had long gone cold. Maggie sat in the high-backed kitchen chair in stunned disbelief. The wood stove was cold to the touch, and the cat was curled into a sleepy ball beside the papers. Maggie couldn't imagine what had triggered the sudden change in him. The menopause had been very hard on her physically and mentally, but it was also apparently devastating for their relationship. The marriage was far from fairytale perfect, but this hit her like a bolt of lightning as she sat there trying to take in and process their conversation before he walked out the front door.

JP had done some research when Maggie began HRT two years ago and was reasonably well-informed when it came to the menopause. It was this research that had him lose heart and faith that Maggie would ever be happy or intimate again. Her treatment was going well, but her attitude had caused him to reach a breaking point. JP had tried many times to build a bridge and was tired of it.

Maggie's first emotion was rage. How dare he falsely accuse her? The sadness was quick to follow and set in hard. She had been going through hell and was told that her bloods were finally good for her stage in the menopause. She didn't feel bad physically any longer, but the internal feelings of judging others constantly, coupled with rage and short-term memory loss, were off the charts. Maggie was shocked awake. The only saving grace she could see at the moment was that the line where JP's signature was supposed to be was blank. He hadn't signed it yet. In a huff, she grabbed a pen and prepared to sign on the line above her name. A lump formed in her throat as her eyes welled up. She began to sob softly and changed her mind. Maggie shuffled them up and put the unsigned documents back into the large envelope.

Over eighteen years ago, Maggie and JP met at a Garda checkpoint on the outskirts of Ashford, County

Wicklow. She had forgotten to put her new tax disc in the car; the old one expired the previous month. JP made her pull over to the hard shoulder in her silver Toyota Corolla.

Maggie pressed the button to roll down her window as JP approached. "You're driving on an expired tax disc, miss," JP informed her.

Maggie flushed with embarrassment. "Ah shite, I have it on my desk at home somewhere. When it arrived, my father had just passed away, and my mind was all over the place. I'm very sorry," she replied.

"I'm sorry for your loss," JP said. "It's no big deal. Present it to the Garda station in Wicklow Town within ten days, and there will be no issues." "You're very good, thanks a million. I'll do it this afternoon," Maggie replied with relief.

As she drove away, Maggie and JP were thinking the exact same thing. They thought they'd both just seen the most attractive person in their lives. When Maggie presented the new disc four hours later, JP was just getting off his shift. He mustered his courage and chanced his arm.

"I see you're all legal now. Fancy a quick coffee? I'm just done with work," JP said with a hopeful smile. "I'd love one," Maggie responded as her heart fluttered. They married a little over a year later. They were both twenty-seven.

As she sat at the kitchen table, unable to think straight, Maggie wanted to ring anyone to have a chat but couldn't. She felt horrible, like a failure, and didn't want anyone to discover what was happening. But, of course, she knew they would find out eventually if she didn't fix the situation. Thinking about who she would call if she could, Maggie realised there wasn't anyone in her friend circle she was close to anymore.

Maggie had always been a very easy-going and carefree

person. She would be the first to lend a sympathetic ear to a needy friend and always put others first. Her social group used to be expansive and diverse; she was close to her friends and family. Slowly, imperceptibly, there had been a shift she hadn't noticed. Her doctor was excellent and suggested she begin HRT sooner rather than later. Maggie shared her early experiences with JP, but realised now that she hadn't spoken to him about anything relating to her transition for well over a year. Was this related to what he was referring to when he suggested that she *have a long, hard think about how she had treated him and her friends the past two years?*

The past three years had been challenging, and the HRT was only making the menopause bearable. Her personality had dramatically shifted, and she was no longer carefree or attentive to others' needs. It was for this reason that she had nobody to ring. She had effectively ostracised every one of her friends in one way or another over what she now recognised as very minor and petty stuff. However, every situation seemed massive to her for some strange reason at the time. The more she reflected, the deeper her despair grew.

Maggie poured her cold tea into the sink, filled and boiled the kettle and put a Barry's tea bag in a new cup. She filled a hot water bottle when she finished pouring her cup of tea. She went into the bedroom to have a good cry, cup and bottle in hand, because she wretched. Maggie tucked herself and the almost-too-hot bottle under the covers. She took a small sip of tea and leaned against the pillows to reflect on how her life had gotten to that point. Maggie had always had a large pool of acquaintances and friends, as well as a smaller pool of very close friends. She was sure she could think of at least one friend she could ring when she felt better. Maggie went through them mentally to see who would be the unfortunate soul to help carry her troubles.

Maggie considered the mother of her son's best friend, her former best friend, who was a bookkeeper. They had known each other since the boys were little and had had many coffees together, as well as the occasional girls' night out. Maggie tried to remember the last time they chatted, and it dawned on her that it had been over seven months since they had a falling out. It was a strange period of time on the planet. The governments and media had everyone confused and terrified during the COVID-19 phase. People were divided by fear, ignorance, misunderstanding and mixed messages. Some people followed all the recommendations without question, while others were highly sceptical about the guidelines laid out for everyone to follow. It was utter chaos on a planetary scale. The more the two talked, the conversation took the form of a debate that became fairly heated. Throw in the fact that she was having a horrible day with a nauseating period, and they both said things they probably regret now. However, the fallout from the lockdowns, the pandemic, and the menopause had likely permanently ended that friendship.

The next person that popped into her head was her childhood friend. They grew up as next-door neighbours and were bridesmaids for each other at their weddings. But, like the bookkeeper, it had been many months since they last had pleasant words. And, like the bookkeeper, the falling out happened on a day that she shouldn't have even gotten out of bed due to her crippling menstrual pain. Maggie remembered being like a honey badger bitten by a cobra. Her friend was having marital problems, and Maggie didn't pay attention or even pretend to care what her friend was saying. Maggie couldn't recall precisely what was said in the exchange, but her friend lost her temper at Maggie's total lack of concern, and when her friend left the coffee shop, she said never to speak to her again. Maggie hadn't and now couldn't. She was stunned by the two recollections. Her behaviour terminated both friendships.

Maggie tried to go to sleep, curled around her hot water bottle like the cat on the kitchen table. Sleep wouldn't come, and she once again tried to decide whom she would ring up to meet for a chat, a rant, and maybe a cry. Maggie thought of her sister but quickly dismissed the idea. The falling out occurred on the day of a protest in Belfast. Maggie hadn't slept the previous night. The arrogant agitators, screaming and yelling obscenities, really got under her sleepless skin. She had an awful headache. Maggie was in a positively foul humour. Her sister was always quick-tempered and was having none of Maggie's sass when they met up. Her sister didn't have any trouble going through the menopause, so she was clueless about what was happening to Maggie. This, deep down, had always pissed Maggie off.

"Maggie, would you ever just cop the fuck on? This is a serious protest," her sister said at a loud volume.

"Excuse me?" Maggie said in a voice at a volume higher than necessary. "You haven't a clue what I'm going through, you had it easy compared to what is happening to me."

"Do you actually think that?" her sister asked sharply as her volume ratcheted up a notch. "We all go through it, you're just softer than me, you always were," her sister jabbed.

This verbal punch was the last straw and Maggie snapped as her switch was tripped. "You can fuck right off, I'm serious, FUCK OFF!"

Maggie screamed back louder than intended. She was satisfied when her sister did precisely that, turning on her heels and made her way to the other side of the crowd of women's supporters. That's the last time they chatted. Her sister wouldn't even answer the phone or return texts. Another bridge burned. When departing any conversation, Maggie realised she had been throwing matches over her shoulder for the past year.

Maggie rolled over and picked up her phone. The time was 23:23. She usually considered numerical patterns as good omens and smiled to herself. She considered ringing her husband to see if there was a chance he was regretting his actions, but decided not enough time had passed for him to properly miss her and realise the error of his ways. Maggie scrolled through Facebook and clicked on her 'friends' list to see if there was anyone she could chat with. She got one hell of a shock. The number of friends on her list was less than half of what it was a year ago. There must be some glitch, she thought. Maggie didn't do much on Facebook and couldn't imagine where her friends had gone. Maggie searched for a couple of her better friends and tried to send a friend request and a private message, but found, to her horror, that she'd been blocked. She replayed in her mind the last time she saw each of them. One, Maggie met at Tesco car park. She remembers giving out about the price of petrol and how the government has lost the run of itself. The last time she saw the second friend, Maggie was on a soapbox, talking about the number of illegal immigrants flooding the country. She remembered now always being on a rampage about one thing or another.

Maggie got out of the warm nest of covers, went to the kitchen, poured a large glass of red wine, and returned to bed. As she took her first sip, she deeply reflected on the type of friend she was to her friends. Maggie put the shoe on the other foot and realised that she hadn't been a very pleasant person to be around in the past couple of years. Everything slowly changed over time as she entered a profound and deeper trip into the menopause. In her mind, Maggie was the same person she'd always been. Instead of communicating with her friends, she habitually listened to the news morning, noon, and night. The toxic media had now shaped her life narrative. Maggie had to face the fact that she not only wasn't the same, and she wouldn't want to be friends with someone like herself. Maggie now understood that it wasn't Facebook that had the glitch; it was, in fact, her. The tears began to well up slowly at this realisation, and when the first tear hit her lip, she tasted the saltiness with the tip of her tongue, and the floodgates opened. Maggie wailed in anguished tears and felt like a truly horrible human being. She now knew she'd been in denial over her actions, and this was a hard pill to swallow. Before the menopause, she was a kind and very calculated conversationalist, but now she was angry all the time and didn't realise it. Life was normal in her reality. The reality she was creating for those around her was very uncomfortable. She drifted off to a very fitful night's sleep.

The following day, Maggie woke, showered and made a cup of tea to think about what she would do next. She opened the *Find My Phone* app and nervously clicked on the thumbnail that would locate JP's phone. She was terrified the blue dot would be in a housing estate somewhere, and her husband was with another woman, one who was more likeable and at least honest with herself. The blue dot was at the Iveagh Hotel in Dublin. She felt equal parts relief and panic. He wasn't at a house with someone but at a hotel. Was he with someone there? Maggie wanted to ring to discuss her epiphany about the kind of person she'd been and tell him that she would get professional help to deal with her denial, attitude, and actions. She couldn't.

Maggie thought long and hard. She took several deep breaths and carefully worded a WhatsApp message. She read it, re- read it and changed it several times, unsure she even wanted to send it, terrified of the reply. Maggie wanted it to be perfect. She pressed send and her stomach dropped when she saw the two grey check marks appear indicating that it had been successfully received: *'I'm very sorry for how I have treated you and everyone close to me the past couple of years. I had blocked out all the horrible things I had done and said. The divorce papers physically shook me out of the slumber of denial, and all the ways I'd been mean and hurtful came flooding back last night. Is there a chance we can work this out, love?'*

Maggie hoped for an immediate reply; however, a full day passed, and the grey check marks hadn't turned blue. Therefore, it was an unread message. Fear and panic set in, and it was genuine. She imagined all the different situations that prevented JP from even reading the message. All the scenarios centred around some woman he was with. She must be kinder, probably better-looking and definitely younger. Maggie and JP were the same age. He wouldn't want another woman in the menopause in his life. Maggie was now desperate, but still couldn't ring him. She was thinking of him having dinner with another woman. If his phone rang, he'd probably not answer it in front of her. No, she couldn't ring him. Maggie decided on another message: *'I see you haven't seen my message. I love you and hope you're well. If there's any chance you're willing to talk with me, I'm totally ready. I'm soooooooooo sorry. I really love you. Please message me back.'* She read it three times, then pressed the Send button.

Maggie woke up early the next morning and immediately checked her phone. The four check marks on the messages were still grey. Both of her messages remained unread. She was in between rage and panic. What if he's distracted by someone else? What if we are really done as a couple? Maggie clicked on his contact details and almost rang him. But she stopped herself. If she spoke to him, she might say something that would be the last words ever spoken between them. Instead, she checked the *Find My Phone* app again. He was still at the same hotel. She sent another message: '*Please read and reply. I'm ready to try anything to make this work. Can you at least just say something?*' She pressed Send, and immediately, all six checkmarks turned blue. He'd read them all at the same time. The *reply bubbles* on the bottom of her screen meant JP was typing. Her heart was racing like a greyhound after a trip around the track. The reply was only two words. Maggie broke down in tears of relief immediately. There was hope, and they were going to do it together. The reply simply said: 'MARRIAGE COUNSELLING.'

RICH MAN BROKE

Ryan was the only child of two very cool parents who ensured his life was what any kid would dream of. They owned a local business that did an excellent trade, so he and his parents took as many holidays as possible. His parents' first and last holiday without him was in Spain. A local bus driver ploughed into their rented Harley-Davidson as he was texting. They were tragically killed on impact. Ryan was just twenty-four years old. He was now the owner of a successful business and a mortgage-free home, but he was alone. They all lived in Cork, and any family he had was in Dublin. He considered selling everything and moving closer or anywhere away from the constant reminders of his incredible parents. Fiona walked into Ryan's shop and approached him behind the counter.

"Do you, by chance, know how to change a tyre? I've tried it myself, but the nuts seem to be stuck," Fiona blurted. His shop had nothing to do with automotive supplies, so the question confused and amused him.

"I do indeed know how to change a tyre; I'll help you if I can," Ryan answered as he reached for his keys and the *closed* sign for the door.

They walked a short distance to a car park. Ryan couldn't help but smile. The small force of nature striding along next to him talked nonstop.

"I must be the unluckiest person alive. This is typical for a normal day in my life," Fiona rambled. "I'm going to be late for the wedding; I just know it. I'm late for everything. My Da says I'll even be late for my own funeral. I kinda hope he's right about that," she laughed.

Ryan walked in silence as there was no break in her chatter. He was laughing inside at the constant barrage of banter she was spouting. "Here she is," Fiona said, pointing to a very clean black Micra with a flat back tyre. The car and her hair were the same colour, and both were shiny for the wedding day that was in it.

Ryan opened the boot, retrieved the jack, lug wrench and spare tyre, and set to work as fast as possible. He couldn't explain why, but he thought this little firecracker of energy was one incredible person.

With considerable effort, the tyre was changed in less than fifteen minutes. Fiona talked behind him the entire time. He found out she was a bridesmaid in a few hours. She was a local attending Cork University. She was studying accounting. They were the same age. She lived with her parents, which is why she was single, she said. He had never heard someone talk so much without taking a breath.

He snapped the cover back on the wheel and stood to face her. They made the first real eye contact since the adventure began. She stopped talking immediately. "Well, there ya are, yer good to go," Ryan said, giving her a quick wink.

"God, that was so fast. You're just the best. You must come to the afters party at the hotel," she rattled off like an auctioneer. Ryan laughed and accepted on the spot. "I'll see you in a few hours," he said. His hands were filthy, so they nodded and planned to meet at the hotel.

Ryan walked back to his shop feeling better than he had since the accident and looking forward to seeing Fiona soon. He finished the end-of-day work early and put the closed sign on the door.

Then, he walked the short distance home to prepare for his first social interaction since his parents' deaths. Ryan found himself smiling for the second time that day. Fiona certainly had a positive effect on him. As he dressed, Ryan began to wonder how much or how little about his life he could share with her. He was wealthy on paper, and the shop had to hire additional staff after the accident due to the community's support. He would never have to worry about money, making him an attractive partner. He decided just to play it by ear and see how the night unfolded.

The reception was packed. Fiona saw him walk into the room before he saw her. "RYAN, OY, over here," she yelled loudly over the DJ music, then waved for him to come to the head table.

She was obviously enjoying herself. "Everyone, this is Ryan, my knight in shining armour." She had told everyone the story, and they all said fair play for helping. The groom said if anyone needed help, she did, and everyone laughed. They drank and danced, taking frequent breaks to get some fresh air outside. That's when they would learn more about each other. On their last trip outside, he decided to ask her out for a proper lunch or dinner so they could just chat. He simply dove straight to the point. "Fancy dinner on Friday night?" Ryan asked. "Oh, thank God, if you weren't going to ask, I was. I'd love dinner," Fiona said in a relieved tone.

Following dinner on their fifth official date, Ryan asked if she would like to come to his house for a drink and maybe watch a movie. Fiona smiled and gladly accepted. They held hands as they made their way back. Once inside the house, she stopped and then slowly turned in a circle. His house looked like a typical semi-detached house on the outside. Inside was a different story. The back extension was designed to resemble a rustic cottage over 100 years old, complete with a wood-burning stove. The rest of the house was a blend of state-of-the-art mod-cons and very rustic antiques. It didn't look like a house a lad in his twenties would live in, but he loved his parents' style, stating he wouldn't ever change a thing. A whole year passed in the blink of an eye.

As a newly certified accountant, Fiona began handling all the accounts at the shop and even managing the staff, so Ryan could focus on running the business properly. He hadn't realised how hard he had been working until she came along to pick up some slack. Fiona was a natural in business and management. She stayed at his gaff most nights but hadn't *officially* moved in. In fact, they hadn't talked about it yet. The arrangement for her to work at the shop and semi-move into the house seemed to simply happen. Ryan was grateful, but her little touches here and there around the house didn't seem to fit the theme. Fiona liked Ikea, and he loved the rustic feel. It was no big deal, though. Another twenty-one years passed.

They had been married for twenty years and had two young children, but they waited several years before starting a family to focus on the business. They were in a very comfortable financial position. Ryan had a young lad managing the shop now, and Fiona was a very shrewd investor.

Ryan remembered being worried on their first date about saying too much to women because of gold diggers, but she had done the opposite. It took her a while to convince him to part with his savings, but he changed his mind when he saw what she could do with it. Fiona had tripled their savings in ten years, and the dividends would take care of them for the rest of their lives. They would have a mini financial empire to hand down to their two kids.

The marriage was happy most of the time. Following the birth of their second child, Fiona never regained any lasting passion. Like most newlyweds, they used to be very active in the bedroom in the early days, but they rarely made love now, and it was always very quick if they did. This scenario went on for a few years, and then her moods began to match her attitude in the bedroom. Fiona was very quick to anger and never wanted any type of physical contact. They were a socially active couple and would attend many events. Everyone who looked at them was envious of their station in life. Nobody had any idea behind closed doors; there was nothing to envy in the bedroom.

The house had changed a fair bit over the years, but the rustic theme was still dominant. Ryan knew Fiona would prefer a different style, but they agreed to keep it the same as his parents'. It was his parents who allowed them to have the life they lived. Fiona occasionally mentioned that his parents gave them a start, but she built it into what it is. He didn't particularly care to hear that. She was changing inside, but the world around her remained stagnant. Fiona knew she had to do something, anything, to facilitate a change in her reality to maintain her sanity. She feared becoming consumed by boredom and fading into invisibility if she maintained the status quo.

Ryan had to leave for a four-day trade show in London to restock their shop. He'd taken the same trip four times a year since they became a couple. They always had a romantic night before he left, and he was looking forward to it because of the long dry spell in their intimacy. It didn't happen. Fiona said something about a property investment she needed to sort out, and she'd be in bed later. It was much later, and Ryan was fast asleep.

After being away for four days, Ryan returned late in the afternoon and arrived home to a major construction site. There were two massive skips full of many of their household items, along with a digger and a shipping container in the garden. He got out of the cab and stood motionless in his driveway, looking at the carnage. Ryan took ages to anger, but rage surfaced immediately, and he stormed into the home, which he no longer recognised. It was now a modern-looking house. Ryan had no idea how they'd done everything so fast, but the changes they'd made inside were irreversible. He was raging and only briefly made eye contact with his wife. Fiona smiled hopefully, but her expression changed when she saw he didn't like the change. She was changing on the inside and desired to reflect that on the outside. Ryan stormed into the bedroom and changed clothes. He took running shoes out of the bottom of the wardrobe that he'd only tried on but never run in. Ryan didn't say a word as he passed her on his way out the front door for his first-ever run. He just couldn't believe what she'd done. Ryan had no idea what running people even did. Having no idea where he was going, Ryan knew he must run away from what he had just arrived at. He managed to get to the end of the street before stopping to catch his breath, having run only about 200 metres. He crouched over with his hands on his knees and reflected on the disaster he'd just run away from. Ryan was breathing heavier than he had in years. It felt horrible. The style of the house now betrayed the spirit of his late parents. He was overwhelmed by a combination of anger and sadness, and knew there was no turning back the clock, as the items in the skip were mostly destroyed. Ryan was a wealthy man financially, but he was crippled in spirit.

Ryan knew his wife had behaved differently in the past few years, but this was just crazy stuff in his mind. He sat on a park bench for at least half an hour, trying to decide what he would do or say when he got home. He got up and very slowly ran back home. He was sweaty and went straight into the shower. All the lights in the house were off, so he knew the kids were asleep. He didn't care if he woke her up when he opened their bedroom door. He couldn't believe what he was looking at once again. Their room wasn't massive, but it had always been very comfortable. She'd somehow managed to get a super king-sized bed into the room while he was out for his run. There was only a small path to walk to the dressers and wardrobes that just about opened. He was about to say something. However, Ryan held his tongue. He wasn't sure he could control what might come out if he said anything. He was exhausted from travel, turmoil and the run. He went to sleep; hopeful things would be better in the morning.

Ryan continued his nightly runs, and Fiona continued to make changes to the house. He simply accepted that his life was now ruled by a person who made a lot of money but had no passion for intimacy or compassion for his feelings. He remembered his past love life as he piled on the miles every night. Running became his new passion. He joined not one but two running clubs. Each met at different times on different days. Ryan became a running fanatic and started participating in official races. He completed three 10K races before building up the courage to attempt his first half-marathon. He was intoxicated with running and was able to forget the stuff at his parents' home, which was now hers. It wasn't his. He barely recognised anything when he was there. It was like living in a perpetually changing Airbnb.

Ryan's fifth official marathon was the day before the family's Spanish holiday. He'd run faster than ever and was in the shape of his life. His belly was flat, and his body was flexible because he stretched every night in the new modern conservatory. He was getting used to the house's layout and even said as much to her. He knew he was lying, but he needed to break the ice to become close again, possibly. They both kept fit, and he still fancied her.

The family arrived at their villa; the children full of excitement for the days ahead. The kids had gone to the pool, and she was getting changed in the loo. He was already in his swim trunks and craving her. He gently pressed the loo door open as she put her top on. He saw her left breast for the first time in over a year.

Fiona yelled. "Keep the bloody door closed," she said as she covered herself. "I need some privacy here," she said as she pulled the door shut.

He was a rich man, but he was broke.

A WALK TO THE RIVER

Gareth found himself at a rural Garda station. The chair he sat on was old, cold, and made of metal. He shifted a bit to try to find any comfort. He knew he looked as agitated on the outside as he felt on the inside. He was grief-stricken and heartbroken, but he was going to do what was asked of him. He was cut from a cloth composed of parish and family responsibility. Gareth ran his massive hand through his thin, greying hair and shifted in the chair again. He crossed his blue jean-covered ankles as he looked down at his old, worn, sturdy farm boots. He raised his eyes for an instant and then looked down at his hands in his lap. They were rugged and calloused hands from a lifetime on the family farm. And no matter how much he washed them, the fingernails always seemed to have a line of dirt at the tips of each nail.

Garda Doyle took out a notepad and pen. He clicked the pen into action as chair legs screeched on the floor from another room. The cup of steaming tea gave off a soothing smell. The Garda solemnly stated, "I'm sorry we have to do this, but it's necessary to follow standard procedure. Now, tell me what you know about what happened to Niamh."

Gareth clasped his thick fingers together and quietly cleared his throat as he looked up again. This time, he didn't look back down. He was ready to tell his story. His sad eyes matched his weak smile as he cleared his throat again and began speaking. Garda Sergeant Doyle was well known in the area. He and Gareth had chatted many times over the years.

"Well, I first saw Niamh at a GAA match between our parishes. It was at my club," he quietly began.

"That's the same way I met my missus," Garda Doyle said.

Gareth continued, "I remember it was lashing out of the Heavens and by halftime, the pitch was a soggy mess. We only glimpsed each other through the sheets of rain, but we both knew we'd seen one another. I'd never really given a second thought about girls. Everything from her hair to her eyes and the hurley in her hand had caught my attention. She was beautiful to me. We were sixteen years old."

Garda Doyle shook his head slightly as he said, "We were the same age as yourselves."

Gareth explained, "The next summer was a game of cat and mouse between obligations on the farm, and trying to *accidentally on purpose* see her. I drove the tractor into town more often than necessary to possibly catch a glimpse of her walking with her friends on the main street. She was easy to spot from a distance. She was a bit taller than her friends and walked in a particular and determined way. But it was her bright auburn hair that hung long and straight down her back to her waist that was the beacon my eyes always noticed first. When that happened, on a rare occasion, we both smiled at each other, and I felt incredible for the rest of the day. I worked with my heart full of joy following an *accidental* encounter. Nothing could dampen my spirit on those days. I would return to the farm and take on the worst jobs after a sighting, because I was on a high like no other. Even mucking out the pig shed was enjoyable. This *horse-play* lasted about two years until we were eighteen."

The sergeant smiled and agreed, "Her long red ponytail hanging out of her helmet, down the back of her jersey on the pitch used to give my missus bad dreams. They were friends off the pitch, but sworn enemies on it"

Gareth gave a weak laugh and resumed his story. "We

formally became a couple at her club's annual GAA dinner dance. The clubhouse was completely decked out in red and green flags with three disco balls hung from hooks in the ceiling. There was no chance in hell that we would announce our intentions to be together at my club. The slagging I would get from the lads would be relentless and spoil the night." The Garda laughed and agreed, "That's always the way, so."

Gareth recalled, "The evening was magical in every way. We ate good food, drank a few pints of Guinness, and clapped for the award recipients. Niamh collected Camogie Player of the Year, and all eyes were on us when she returned to their table."

Gareth continued, "I remember like it was yesterday, I was delighted for her, but equally happy for myself to be her date. Then it was time for the DJ. The long tables were cleared of the teacups, pint glasses, plates and cutlery. The hurling lads quickly folded and stacked the tables against the wall where they were always kept. The house lights dimmed, and green and red stage lights pointed at the small, bald middle-aged DJ. There was a blast from a smoke machine, which clouded the room and made the reflections from the disco balls shine like tiny torches all around the room. He kicked the party off with a lively Christy Moore tune and a few Dubliners tunes for the mature members before blasting another plume of smoke and launching into YMCA. That song got everyone up dancing; the rest of the night belonged to the younger members.

We danced the night away and shared our first kiss at the end of the evening around the side of the clubhouse." Gareth paused for a moment to savour the memory before speaking again. "We spent the entire next year together as much as possible. She would occasionally come to the farm to help with the chores so we could spend time together. Even stacking itchy hay bales in the barn loft was fine so long as we were together. Nothing felt like work when she was there. We laughed at the same things at the same time and seemed to know what the other was thinking. In my mind, we were destined to be together forever. But what happened last week proved me wrong. We didn't have an easy early life, but life was grand once we overcame a few rough patches. Niamh seemed to drift away from life for the past few years until she disappeared. I really don't know what else to say."

While the two men knew each other, the interview was far more than a simple formality. The Garda had thought he'd know people in the past, only to be shocked by what happened behind closed doors. He told Gareth this phase of the interview was over and would be in touch as the investigation moved forward.

Gareth nodded once and stood slowly. The chair screeched as it slid backwards on the cold concrete floor. He turned, his head hanging low, and walked towards the door.

"Take care, Gareth. If there is anything I can do for you, don't hesitate to ask, and if you can think of anything to help, please get in touch," Garda Doyle said to his back. Gareth turned his head halfway around and in a low, slow voice replied, "Thanks."

GARETH AND NIAMH

Shortly before they turned nineteen, Niamh came to the farm. It was the middle of summer and the beginning of the GAA Championships. Gareth had fanciful thoughts dancing in his head about lifting the county final trophy daily and was sure Niamh's club would do the treble. The sun was splitting the stones, and the coconut smell of the gorse shrub's yellow blossoms around the farm perimeter was intoxicating. Gareth saw Niamh coming up the drive, and his heart skipped a beat as it always did whenever he saw her. But something was wrong this time. She wasn't prancing up the lane like a show pony as usual. She was doing quite the opposite. He noticed she was visibly shaken and upset as she staggered towards him. There were dirty streaks on her cheeks from what must've been hours of tears.

Gareth dropped the chain on the gate, making a loud clang that startled the chickens beneath his feet in all directions. He sprinted the short distance and embraced her tightly in his dirty, sweaty farm boy arms. He didn't ask her what was wrong. He didn't have to. Deep in his soul, he felt he knew what the trouble was. He had been worried for a good while, too. They had only *been together* a few times when the passion took over, but they didn't know how to prevent pregnancy. This was rural Ireland. People didn't talk about stuff like that.

They were alone on the farm except for the livestock, but they walked into the haybarn and climbed the old wooden ladder affixed to the far wall up into the dusty loft to sit on the bales the pair had stacked together last season. They hadn't been passionate yet when they'd arranged those bales into neat stacks, and Gareth wished like mad that they could go back to that day and make different choices. But somehow, strangely, he didn't have any regrets. He knew he loved Niamh with all his heart. He was numb and dumbfounded, but she was uncontrollably hysterical. She would weep quietly, then scream in rage and pound her fists on her legs so hard he was sure she'd hurt herself. He tried to hug her, but she pushed him firmly away and threw herself into his arms the next instant. She was a mess. Niamh finally took several deep breaths and leaned back against an itchy bale. They held each other's hands, and he looked at her. She was beautiful, even with tear-soaked eyes and messy hair. But she looked so very young at that moment. And he thought to himself that he barely had to shave once a fortnight. They were too young for this to be happening.

During this era of rural Catholic Ireland, there were no options other than childbirth. You were having it, and that's final. Once they accepted what was going to happen, they were smart enough not to wait too long before setting off the atom bombs in their respective houses. If they were old enough to make a baby, they decided to take whatever consequences might follow. They had no idea how dire those consequences would be, but they could've never imagined that both families deciding to fly Niamh to Australia to live with her aunt and uncle would be the agreed-upon option. The plan was for them not to have contact with each other going forward, and the story down under would be that Niamh's husband was killed in a freak farming accident. It was an utterly unbelievably cruel plan. Niamh and Gareth were too shocked to say anything.

Niamh spent three long days in her room crying, sleeping and then getting fits of rage and hysterics. Gareth missed her terribly, but he could do nothing to help her. He remembered a year ago when she would do something like this every couple of months, and there would be a few very touchy days, but everything would be grand soon enough. During those few tense days, she seemed to act like a completely different person. He never asked about it. This was rural Catholic Ireland, and nobody talked about anything like that.

Gareth was understandably obsessing over their predicament. He made a massive decision. He had been quiet and working harder on the farm than ever to distract his worried mind, but he now knew the course of action he must take. Gareth was never one to rock the boat, but he was prepared to sink the ship if they sent Niamh away. He told his family that if she were shipped off to Australia, he would do anything to go to her as soon as possible and never return to the farm. He truly meant it. This was the first time Gareth had said anything about his feelings in the situation. Nobody had asked him, and of course, he kept quiet because they had done such a horrible thing in his mind. But Gareth raised his voice to a shout and pounded his meaty fist on the kitchen table when he vowed to move abroad. His shocked mum and dad understood that he was deadly serious, and they knew the farm would fail without him. They tried for a minute to talk him around to their way of thinking, but Gareth was having none of it. He stood tall at the table with his arms crossed over his chest and kept shaking his head no. He was an adult, they had done an adult thing, and he was making an adult decision.

Left with no options, the two families got together again, and the plans quickly changed. The farm was far more important than the negative optics of a young married couple in the eyes of their friends and neighbours. A small but comfortable caravan was set up on the farm in a secluded area surrounded by shade trees. Niamh moved into it the day they were married in a quiet civil ceremony at the registry office. There would be no grand Catholic wedding, like everyone had imagined only a few short months ago, if they were to marry eventually. Gareth felt happy for the first time in a long time. He had his young wife, a growing baby in her belly and the farm. He went to work to make the best of this situation.

Their first visit to the doctor was, unfortunately, highly uncomfortable for the young couple. The doctor was an older man and didn't hide the fact that he wasn't impressed with their ages or how they went about getting married. They both knew this was going to get harder and harder as her belly grew, but the first visit was over. Holding hands, they crossed the road from the clinic and climbed up the three steps into his tractor cab to drive home. Niamh sat on the armrest beside him for the slow, bumpy trip home. Gareth had failed his driving test, so he wasn't allowed to drive a car yet. Niamh had her test coming up, so they were hopeful they could drive to the next appointment in a car, rather than a tractor.

Niamh took driving lessons from her uncle, who was an excellent teacher and sympathetic to her situation. He was a *surprise* birth thirty-four years earlier and knew the hell his parents went through in the early days of their forced marriage. They chatted constantly during the lessons, and Niamh always felt reassured when the lesson ended. As hoped, she passed her test on the first go and was over the moon. Gareth climbed into the passenger seat of her uncle's borrowed car. Niamh drove them both to their six-month checkup. They went to a different doctor in the city, instead of the one in the village, hoping for a better experience this time. It was better in some ways, but ultimately far worse.

The young doctor was much more sympathetic than the old lad was. He had seen many couples in their situation and was non-judgmental towards them. He had all the modern equipment in his office at the hospital and was very professional. Ultrasound scans were only new in Ireland, but were part of the healthcare system, so they decided to have one done. Niamh lay on the paper-covered table and pulled her loose shirt up. The nurse squirted a cold, clear gel onto her growing belly, and the doctor used a wand with a metal disc on the tip to spread the gel around. He looked up at the screen, preparing to point out the various parts of the developing baby's body. His demeanour changed in an instant. The results were catastrophic. The doctor's eyes widened when he stared at the monitor. What he said next was cataclysmic. There was no sign of any spinal formation. Gareth asked what that meant.

The doctor cleaned the gel off and hung the wand on its hook. He slowly turned to face them as the nurse used tissues to wipe the gel off Niamh's belly. He took a deep breath and donned a very sombre expression as he slowly shook his head. He explained there was no chance of a live birth. Niamh sat up as she pulled her top down over her belly, which now held no hope for life. She was so stunned that she couldn't say a word and staggered out of the clinic in a zombie-like daze. She made it to the car before the reality of the diagnosis finally hit her like an avalanche. She let out a banshee-like, blood-curdling scream and collapsed onto the ground in a heap in front of the car. Gareth scooped her up in his arms and tried to comfort her, but he was reeling just as much as she was. He wanted to say everything would be okay, but he knew nothing was okay about this situation. Instead, he simply muttered that they would get through this together. Even though he didn't have a licence, he was a good driver, so he drove them back to the farm.

Abortion was not an option, of course, so it was going to be a horrific waiting game for everyone. The reality of the impending end of the saga was the only thing Niamh thought about. One month later, a spontaneous abortion occurred. Niamh cried for her loss and felt a mix of relief and sadness at the same time. This dichotomy of emotions and the sudden hormonal changes had her going through episodes of grief, guilt and rage again as she barely came out of their tiny bedroom for the next week. She beat her fists on her legs so hard that she left bruises like she'd been hit with a hurley. Gareth worried about how she punished herself, but they never really talked about it.

Eventually, her friends from the GAA club came to the rescue. Gareth was never so grateful to anyone. They rallied around her for several days like mother hens. They cooked and cleaned the caravan and took walks with her to have the chats. Two women, who had been through similar experiences, talked about it for a change. Niamh had known them for years but hadn't a notion they'd been through a similar hell that she had gone through. That probably helped the most as she didn't feel alone anymore. Gradually but steadily, she returned to herself and began living life again like she used to. She even resumed playing camogie and was more impressive than ever on the pitch. It was as if she was taking her rage out on the sliotar and the opposition, rather than herself. She admitted that she wouldn't be playing if she had a newborn to look after and felt conflicting emotions about this. Life was definitely getting better.

The next several years saw them settle into rural farm life, immersed in the GAA. They both played for their clubs, but they also began training and coaching the youth players. Niamh was very good on the farm and brilliant with the young players she was coaching. They started talking about having children of their own. Many of their friends were starting families and were of a proper age now to try again. Their only real problem was that Niamh would experience debilitating menstrual cycles. Niamh would not leave the house and would spend most of the day in bed. She would miss training, farm chores and coaching the young kids. It was so bad one weekend that she missed a semifinal match, which they thankfully won without her.

By the time they were twenty-five, most of their friends had children, and they had been trying but were having trouble for some reason. They couldn't understand how it accidentally happened so easily the first time, and it couldn't happen again when they knew what they were doing. Twice the pregnancy test was positive, only for her to lose the baby a month or two later. She began to get very depressed and seemed to lose hope. The week before her thirtieth birthday, Niamh had a positive pregnancy test again. She didn't tell anyone except Gareth this time. The crushing grief and accompanying form of embarrassment when she lost the babies was overwhelming, and she didn't want to go through it again. It was their secret. The weeks turned into months, and finally, six months passed. It was now apparent to everyone that they were having a baby…finally.

They were actually having twins, much to their shock. When the doctor put the gel-covered wand on her, he pointed out the two very obvious bodies developing. And everything looked perfect. Relief flooded them. They were nervous wrecks heading into the appointment, fearing the same fate as last time. With nothing to worry about, life on the farm took on a happy air. Niamh was glowing and growing. She did her work as usual until she couldn't. Gareth was strutting around like a show bull anticipating the arrival of their kids.

The last few months of her pregnancy were very difficult. Niamh experienced nearly every difficulty in the book. She had rancid heartburn and was nauseous all the time. Niamh had low back pain and pain in the front of her pelvis. She had two very worrying days where she thought she would lose them because of a spot of blood, but everything was fine. The doctor decided to schedule a C-section since she had so much trouble during the pregnancy and had to rest in the last month. Everything went smoothly from then on.

By the time the twins were ten years old, Niamh was the cornerstone of her GAA club, and they were the centre of her universe. She still had terrible issues every few months, but since she had the twins, she didn't go as deep into the depression on the days that were very bad because she had them to look after. As for what the twins thought about those days, well, they were normal to them. They were just mum's quiet days.

At age fifteen, the twins were a great help on the farm and were stars on the GAA pitch. Niamh stopped coaching and did less at the club. She seemed to become quieter. Many evenings, she would take a walk to the riverbank at the bottom of the farm. It wasn't a particularly big river. It made peaceful babbling sounds as she sat surrounded by tall grasses, nettles and thistles. Once every couple of years, the rains would be heavy enough for it to burst its banks. It would be a raging torrent for a few days then. The currents would pull anything underwater that was unfortunate enough to end up in the river. During those times, nobody was allowed near it. The twins never went near it, and the livestock instinctively avoided it; both were good that way. The walks became frequent enough over the years that Niamh had worn a well-trodden path in the tall grasses leading to the bank.

The eighteenth birthday party for the twins was planned a whole month in advance because the family was now local GAA royalty. It would be a fabulous disco-type party with beer and tent camping on the farm for some of their friends. On the morning of the party, Niamh mentioned to Gareth that they didn't have kids anymore; they had young adults. She seemed sad, but he was proud that they had raised two beautiful children who were an asset to the farm, the parish, and the planet. Niamh was quiet all day, and instead of joining in the celebrations for the evening, she stayed only long enough to sing the song and have some of the impressive cake she had made. She then disappeared. She spent most of the evening on the riverbank.

When Niamh turned fifty, she realised her zest for life was gone. She hadn't been in the GAA club for a couple of years and didn't seem like herself. Her brain didn't seem to work like it used to. She was absent-minded and forgetful frequently. Niamh would be sad one day and angry the next, and she was like a furnace in bed, sweating, so there was no chance of intimacy. That seemed to have slowed down in the past few years and never returned. Niamh didn't talk to anyone, and when Gareth suggested a visit to a doctor, she simply shook her head and went for a walk to the riverbank.

The days on the farm seemed like a routine affair for the following year. Niamh seemed a shell of what she once was the day she turned fifty-one. It had rained heavily for two days, and the river had burst its banks as usual. Niamh saw the twins that morning and had a good breakfast with them. They chatted for an unusually long time about their childhood and growing up on the farm. The twins had splurged and bought her a stylish new raincoat and wellies with a flower pattern for her birthday present. Niamh kissed them both and told them how proud she was of them. Fostering a forlorn feeling, she put on her new coat and boots and said she was going for a walk. The well-worn path to the riverbank was the last footsteps she ever took.

There was a missing person's report filed, and for a very short time, before the Garda interview, Gareth was considered a suspect in Niamh's disappearance. It was the absolute worst thing he could imagine, but he needed to be strong for the twins, who were now crushed by the loss of their mum. They were all mystified at the death. Boots and a raincoat were found, but no body was discovered. No one could understand what had happened. This was rural Catholic Ireland, and nobody talked about anything like that. It was her last walk to the river.

NOT FAIR

Paul sat in his car with fingers clamped tightly on the steering wheel. His mind was racing in scattered directions. He was at the GAA pitch watching lifelong mates arrive for training. They all looked happy. He felt like he wanted punishment. It was murky, dark and cloudy as the wind gusted. Rain was most definitely on the way at some point during the session. The dreary and heavy weather suited Paul fine because that's precisely where his frame of mind was. The newly installed floodlights cut beams through to the ground as the diesel generator belched smoke to keep them lit. He was still trying to process what had happened earlier that morning at the doctor's appointment with his wife, Maeve. He was awash with disbelief, denial, anger, sorrow and a type of grief. Most of all, Paul felt devastated for his wife. This shouldn't happen to such a beautiful being. It wasn't fair at all. His mum-in-law came over to talk and cry with her daughter. They wanted to be alone, so he figured a hard training session might do him some good. Maeve was 33, and Paul was 31.

They met four years earlier at a mutual friend's barbecue and immediately hit it off. Maeve had just finished her nursing degree, and Paul taught at a local primary school. They found it easy to talk to one another even though they didn't seem to have much in common. He loved solitude and the outdoors, while she preferred activities that involved crowds. Paul was mad about the GAA, and Maeve loved the rugby. As they chatted more, however, they found that their core values and principles aligned with each other's. They both said how much they adored kids and admitted they found each other very attractive. Maeve was 29, and Paul was 27.

They decided that their differences worked well together. Paul found himself at the odd rugby match in the Aviva Stadium and actually enjoyed it. And even though there was no chance of Maeve going wild camping, she occasionally found the peace of glamping lovely. They brought new experiences into each other's lives and found the most crucial ingredient in anything they did was simply the presence of the other. One thing they did have in common was the love of good food. It was at a very posh restaurant in the city centre that Paul proposed, and she accepted. They married a few months later, surrounded by family and close friends. Maeve was 31, and Paul was 29.

Their love for kids led them to start trying as soon as possible. Her nursing knowledge and the regularity of her cycle meant that she knew the optimal time of the month.
"Time to have a go, Paul," Maeve would say.

Paul always laughed at her bluntness and replied, "It would be my pleasure, after you," gesturing toward the bedroom. However, many months passed, and they began to chat about the reality that something wasn't working as it should.
"Something's wrong, Paul, we should be pregnant by now. We need to get to the bottom of this sooner rather than later, we need to see a specialist," Maeve stated. As a nurse, Maeve knew they could be waiting ages for a gynaecologist appointment. "Let's test you first, love, you can get an appointment much quicker," Maeve suggested.

It was only a two-week wait and four days of abstinence leading up to his appointment at a sperm bank in Dublin. Twenty-four hours later, Paul received the results of his sperm motility. The tests revealed Paul was in the higher percentile of fertility. He was relieved, but now the focus shifted to Maeve. And worry began to creep in.

It was a nail-biting three-month wait to see a gynaecologist. They tried each month leading up to the appointment to conceive, but Maeve was beginning to lose hope. She had to admit there was an eerie feeling slithering in that something was seriously wrong. Maeve tried to relax because she was a nurse, and there was no indication anything was amiss other than the fact that she couldn't get pregnant. But that feeling persisted and got much worse, leading up to the day of her exam. It was a comprehensive exam that included a pap smear to check for cervical cancer.

The usual waiting time for pap smear results was about four weeks, and that's what they prepared for. However, after only three weeks to the day, Maeve received an email advising her to contact the doctor's office and schedule an appointment at her earliest convenience. Maeve rang immediately and was in the office the following day. She was told that her pap smear was irregular, and more tests were needed. The eerie feeling returned with a roaring vengeance. Maeve's next stop that same day was the hospital for all the advanced and more thorough tests. They then had to wait again for the results to come back. The worst part was always the waiting.

The wait didn't take long. Only two weeks later, they got into the car to drive to the gynaecologist she'd seen for the initial exam. It was terrible news. Maeve felt sick as she sank into the passenger seat following the appointment, and as Paul closed the car door and put on his seatbelt, he felt panicked.

"We will get through this together, love. You're young, fit, and healthy. We need to try to stay positive," Paul consolingly said as he reached his hand across and placed it on Maeve's knee. "I'm not that young, I am fit, but I'm not healthy. I have cancer," Maeve said in a quiet, breathless voice.

"You know what I mean," Paul replied. "Paul, I need a total hysterectomy, you know that means no children for us. I always imagined a house full of children. That will never happen now," Maeve said as she began to sob.

Paul pulled the VW Golf into a housing estate, found a parking place, and turned the engine off. He opened his door, got out and went around to Maeve's side. He opened her door and helped her to stand facing him. Paul embraced her in his strong arms as she put her head on his chest. "We will get through this. It has nothing to do with children now. Our total focus must be on you and getting you well. We can talk about other options later. Please stay strong, Maeve. I love ya rotten," Paul soothingly said while stroking her hair.

"I love you too," she said. "I'm really scared."

Paul trained like a man possessed that evening as the rain lashed down; he ploughed on. The worse the weather, the better he felt. He couldn't understand how or why this would or could happen to Maeve. It's not fair. Maeve was magnificent in every sense of the word, and now she had to have radical surgery, chemotherapy, and radiation. There was so much information to take in so fast. And he even remembered the word menopause at some point during the whirlwind of consultant meetings. The final part of the training session was the sprints. Paul pushed harder than ever before and was utterly physically exhausted, matching his mental exhaustion. When he got home, his mother-in-law was gone, and his wife was curled up on the sofa in front of a fire that he'd started before he left for training. He took his kit off and snuggled in behind her. Paul was dirty on the outside, and Maeve felt like that on the inside. They had a shower together and went to bed.

The next morning both felt like they could handle the situation, and they vowed to make the best of the shite hand of cards they've been dealt. They met with the specialists who would be looking after Maeve and set out the schedule for the treatments following the operation. There would be adverse reactions to the treatments they were told, so they at least felt forewarned. Their entire focus was on getting through the procedure and the treatments to save her life. Anything said about anything else just kind of went over their heads. When the menopause was mentioned, neither had any questions.

They both just thought it meant that you couldn't have kids.

The operation was flawless, according to the surgeon, and Maeve healed quickly. She was always very fit. With her fitness and age, they were told she should be much better off than the older women who have to go through the same thing. For once, things seemed to be going their way. Maeve sailed through the treatments, and besides losing her hair and being constantly tired, the only other reaction she had was the inability to taste food like she used to. This was a hassle because of their mutual love for good food. When Maeve was finally given the all clear, she had weathered the storm brilliantly. Maeve was 34 and Paul was 32.

The relief of the 'all clear' was immense, and her prognosis was brilliant for her age group. They went out to eat to celebrate as her taste had gradually returned to normal. It was a cool evening, so they wore light jackets for the short walk from the DART station to the restaurant. Maeve's fitness was also beginning to return, but they still sauntered because she would easily get short of breath. The meal was delicious, and they took their sweet time to enjoy it slowly. The food passion was back on, thankfully. While they were waiting for dessert, Maeve suddenly became hot. Very hot.

"Paul, something's wrong. I'm burning up inside and sweating from every pore in my body," Maeve said as she lowered her sweaty head into her soaked palms. "What do you think is going on? Do we need to go to the hospital?" Paul asked in a bit of a panic.

Maeve stood, took off her light jacket, draped it over the back of her chair and said, "I think I just need some fresh air." Paul rushed over to her side, took her arm and slowly helped her outside. Maeve had had many adverse reactions to the treatments and drugs she was on during the cancer treatment. The cocktail of daily tablets she was on had never caused anything like this. Still, it was the only explanation they could think of.

"Let's make an appointment with the specialist and get to the bottom of this love," Paul said. Maeve agreed. They knew there was always a possibility that something could go wrong and feared the worst again. They waited two days to get an appointment with her specialist, and her *dizzy volcano spells*, as she called them, had continued. Not only the spells, but Maeve also began to find herself inexplicably angry at everyone and everything for no reason. This was not normal at all for her. Maeve was glad that she hadn't gone back to work yet. She couldn't imagine dealing with patients. The sudden waves of rage were a new phenomenon. Maeve explained to the specialist what was happening, and some blood was taken. The specialist explained that the new symptoms were most likely her body adjusting to the menopause. She knew she had a tablet for that, so she was confused. Only now did she consider that the early onset caused by her procedure would have to be managed instead of cured.

They were both relieved to find out that it wasn't life-threatening, but they understood that one battle had ended and the next was just beginning. The following year, Maeve closely stuck to the hormone replacement therapy plan. She was now on a tablet, a patch and a gel. She had some good days, but most of that year was a cloud of depression and rage with the odd *dizzy volcano spell* thrown in for good measure. Maeve didn't return to work that year, and she felt grateful that she could concentrate solely on herself.

At the start of her second year on HRT, she saw yet another all-clear of cancer. Maeve's mood began to lift. She felt a bit better on most days. She slept less and got out more on walks, in nature, of all places. They began taking longer walks on forested trails, and she fell in love with the outdoors. They went glamping a few times. Maeve shocked Paul by asking, "Love, can we have a proper wild camping weekend?"

"What? Am I hearing things? I thought you just said you want to go wild camping," Paul mockingly said. Maeve laughed and replied, "With all the changes I've been through, I'm interested in different aspects of life than in the past, and I feel so much peace in nature. "Hell yeah," Paul excitedly replied.

Paul made the site as close to glamping as he could. He started a fire in the round pit of stones as Maeve made herself comfortable on a pad leaning against a log facing the fire. Paul sat beside her, put an arm around her shoulders and pulled her close. The flames danced and darted on the logs as if in celebration of the outcome for the two of them. Both seemed to be lost in a reverie of reflection, surrounded by the scents and sounds of nature. The fire popped and crackled, and the doves roosting in the trees cooed a mournful song. The heady smoke from the birch logs mingled with the intoxicating fragrance of gorse and elderflower, drifting on the gentle currents that floated past. They were silent. Nothing had to be said between them because both knew they had weathered not one but two massive life challenges. Things were going to be grand going forward. This didn't change the fact that they felt what she had to go through was not fair.

FECKIN HIPPIES

Leigh had a very unusual upbringing. He was reared in an extended family of nomadic-type people who travelled from venue to venue, city to city, following a musical band around the USA. It was just as much about the lifestyle as it was about the magical and mystical music. He had no idea what a school was until he was thirteen. His parents were adamant that he was educated as opposed to schooled, so they taught him to read while on the road, and he could write well by age four. His parents were no slouches. Leigh's mum, Karen, was a molecular biologist, and his father, Ralph, used to teach English classes as he travelled the Asian and European continents. He had written two books about his extensive travels.

Leigh's memories of childhood centred around being in a converted school bus, learning as much as possible as fast as possible, and the aromatic smell of cannabis and Nag Champa incense. The music his parents listened to wasn't particularly to his liking, but he loved his life. Leigh had seen The Jungle Book countless times and felt like Mowgli. However, as the years passed, the school bus's magic began to wear off. He started spending more and more time off the bus and said he would like to go to school and travel. His parents were very supportive and suggested that he choose a boarding school, as they would continue their nomadic lifestyle.

Leigh entered high school at age fifteen and was put in with the sophomore class because he was the same age. However, he was quickly moved to the senior class because he seemed like a wizard in all subjects. His homeschooling had him much better educated than the traditional US school system. Leigh graduated first in his class at the age of sixteen and was offered full college scholarships to some of the best universities in the United States. He chose a college in Boston because he loved the autumn when his family was there for the music, and he felt pulled to that particular one for some reason.

Leigh's final year in Boston was also the year he turned twenty-one. He was offered the opportunity in an advanced class on civilisation to travel to Ireland for a three-month stay at University College Dublin, and he felt compelled to take the offer. He found himself saturated in Irish interests for some inexplicable reason. He wasn't a sports fan, but he had always followed the Boston Celtics basketball team, and his favourite college football team was the Fighting Irish of Notre Dame for no particular reason. He felt pulled to the Emerald Island and couldn't wait.

His accommodation for the three-month stay was brilliant. Leigh had a shared student dorm room with two other lads. One was French, Gabriel, and the other was from Cork, Sean. They all got along straight away. The UCD campus was stunning, and the student lifestyle was very laid back. The classes he took during the day only lasted until 3.00 pm, and he always breezed through his assignments, so he had loads of free time to explore and experience Dublin. He loved visiting St. Stephen's Green and walking around the touristy Temple Bar area. He grew up surrounded by people. Therefore, he didn't mind the crowded places. He wasn't shy and mentioned to the lads that they should go out for the night to see if they could meet some women who lived off campus. Leigh had a feeling that he wanted to meet girls who were different from the UCD students he'd met in the past couple of weeks. Sean was adamant they go to a club called Copper Face Jacks, insisting it was the place to *shift* the hottest women, whatever the hell that meant, thought Leigh. It was a foreign country with a foreign language, even though it was English.

Leigh didn't know anything about the GAA, so he had no idea what he was walking into when he entered the disco. A scar-faced bouncer guarded the front door. The featured match that day at Croke Park was a hurling duel between Limerick and Kilkenny, and Coppers was packed. The three lads made their way to the bar and eventually got their pints and scanned the room for a crack or crevasse to stand in. There were many beautiful women, and everyone was pretty well sozzled, but Leigh noticed the women seemed different from most of the girls he'd met at UCD, and he mentioned it to his roommates.

"Leigh, these are *country girls,*" Sean said with pride of county and country. "They come to *the big smoke* for the most important matches in Croke Park and then come to Coppers to meet lads," he finished.

The dance floor was packed as Leigh made his way to the toilet. The queue to get into the women's toilet was massive as usual, and as he walked past it, he briefly made eye contact with a brown-haired girl with dazzling green eyes who smiled at him. She was still waiting for her turn for a pee on his return trip, so he walked straight up to her.

"It's shitty how few toilets there are for women everywhere," Leigh blurted. "My name is Leigh," he said while extending his hand towards her.

She extended her hand in return. "Hiya, I'm Emily. I agree they need loads more toilets for us," she replied. "Are you a Yank or Canadian?" she asked. "I'm American," he said with a laugh. "I'm here studying at UCD for a few months on an exchange programme," Leigh explained. "That's so cool. I love the States and want to go there for a holiday. I could never live there, though. I love Ireland way too much," Emily said. "I'm from Kilkenny, do you know where that is?" she asked."I know it's south of here," Leigh said. "And according to my GAA crazy roommate, they are great at hurling," he added. "They are the best in Ireland," Emily said, beaming with evident pride for her county. "Wait here, it's my turn to wee."

Emily was fascinated with everything about the US, and she was excited to chat more. Leigh laughed at how blunt she was and nodded, "I'll be right here when you're done."

The two of them went for a stroll to get some fresh air and talk without having to shout. Emily was five years older than him and in her last year of medical training to become a general practitioner. This didn't intimidate him at all. He'd always been very mature for his age, and his intelligence was on par with hers, so they got along well immediately.

"I've never been to a doctor," Leigh casually mentioned. Emily stopped strolling and turned sideways to face him. "Sorry, what? Did I hear that right?" she said with confusion etched on her face.

"Yeah, my parents are hippies and they don't trust Big Pharma or people who make money by selling pills to people when they're sick, I was born in a converted school bus in Indiana," Leigh said. Emily laughed nervously and didn't know what to say next. Leigh continued, "I always went along with anything they said when I was a kid, but I think I now understand why they think the way they do."

He explained to her that *healthcare* in the US is profit-driven, so doctors are incentivised to prescribe and treat as much as the private insurance will pay.

Emily nodded and said, "Right, healthcare in Ireland is almost the opposite," she stated. "People can't get the drugs and treatments they need, and the waiting lists for procedures can take years. I want to see if there is a way to improve the system somehow."

It was Leigh's turn to nod. "I don't know a thing about healthcare here, but it can't be as bad as the US. They are pharmaceutical-pushing crazy," he finished.

They sauntered through the damp, narrow cobblestone laneways as they talked about their totally opposite upbringings. They both looked forward to travelling in the future and discovered many desires in common as the minutes devoured the hours. Time seemed to stand still and fly at fast-forward speed simultaneously. The mid-summer sun began to cast rays on the city, and they made plans to have a proper date the following Friday.

Leigh had about two months left in Ireland, and he wanted to spend as much time as possible with the pretty, brown-haired Emily as possible. They began to study together and go out for a meal or pints every chance they had.

When he had only two weeks left, Leigh decided to try to get a good job and move to Ireland. Emily was a major reason, of course, but he also loved the country. Leigh applied to a few firms with his impressive academic resume. He still needed to return to Boston to graduate officially, but that was just a formality. He kept his job applications a secret as he didn't want to get his hopes up and then get crushed, but he had a good feeling. The couple said very sad goodbyes at the departure gate of Terminal 2 at Dublin

Airport, and as they hugged, he whispered that he would see her soon. Emily shot him a puzzled look, but he simply winked and smiled, then went through security.

The morning of graduation from Boston College was three months to the day after he left Ireland. Time, being the trickster it is, made it feel so much longer than the three months he'd spent at UCD. Leigh spoke daily to Emily, and even with the time difference, they managed some pretty steamy Face Timing sessions trans-Atlantic style. He had to get back to Ireland. His parents were in town for the graduation, and he always loved seeing them. Leigh told them all about his long-distance romance with his Kilkenny girl and how she plans to be a doctor. His parents exchanged a worried glance. Leigh quickly explained how much different the Irish medical system was from the US model. They said they understood and ultimately trusted his judgement. His parents were very happy for them both. On the way to the college campus, he checked his emails again. He'd become obsessed since he'd had two Zoom call-back interviews with firms he wanted to work for. Even his parents didn't know about his hopeful plans.

The email from his first-choice job stated that they would be delighted for him to join their firm, offering a generous pay package and covering his relocation expenses to Dublin. They would handle all the visa requirements and requested that he reply as soon as he had made his decision. Leigh couldn't believe it. He'd gotten his dream job, and he got to move to Ireland permanently. He stopped dead in his tracks, and his mom actually bumped into him. She asked if everything was okay. He smugly smiled and spoke every single word out loud for them to hear as he replied his acceptance of the job offer in Ireland. His parents gave a big hoot and hugged him. They couldn't believe he'd kept it a secret. The FaceTime with Emily one minute later was priceless. She broke down in tears, and so did he. Just like that, he couldn't care less about graduation.

Dr. Emily and Leigh lived in a small bungalow in Ballybrack. Over the course of ten years, they had travelled to exactly twenty-five countries together, and their two daughters were with them for eleven. Emily loved doing charity medical work in poorer countries whenever she could, and his job allowed him to work from anywhere that had WiFi. They enjoyed life, and the girls were brilliant little travellers. The kids would often help their mum in the charity clinics. They were young, but both already wanted to become doctors because they viewed the tablets they gave people as magical. They felt like little witches from their favourite books.

Dr. Emily was a general practitioner. However, as she and her patients aged together, she began to find herself trying to manage the symptoms of the menopause in more and more of the women. She was getting good at quickly dialling in what worked the best for each woman. So, as the years passed, and she recognised some of the perimenopause symptoms in herself, she was confident that she would breeze through the transition. After all, she had knowledge, experience, and access to medication, so what could go wrong, she thought.

The first year, her symptoms weren't too bad or unusual, and she didn't need any hormone replacement. Dr. Emily began to exercise more, and she felt more energy, however, her libido had diminished, like many of her patients. She had hot flushes in the evenings, but overall, she was happy with how the menopause was going. As the second year began, she noticed she was having more and more trouble sleeping, and she was angry almost all the time. Her sex drive was non-existent. She knew it was time for the doctor to see a doctor. Her first attempt at a small dose of oestrogen was a disaster.

She had constant headaches, and she knew it was from the patch. They played around with the dosage, but the headaches persisted, so progesterone was added into the mix to see how her body would respond. The response was pretty immediate. She developed a rash on her neck and face and was constantly itchy all over her body. Her mood was going downhill every passing month. Each time she tried a different combination of HRT, the adverse reactions seemed to be worse than the actual symptoms of the menopause. She was constantly arguing with her daughters and Leigh. And nobody was allowed to mention the 'M' word in the house. Dr. Emily felt like a failure.

Leigh was increasingly worried for the past year or so. He watched the most beautiful woman in the world go down a dark hole, and any attempt to talk about it was met with anger and frustration. Desperation was the emotion he was experiencing when he rang his mom in San Francisco to ask if she had any ideas that could help save his wife and marriage. His mom listened carefully for over half an hour without saying a word. Leigh needed to talk to someone, and his mom was an excellent listener who could read his needs very well. As he spoke, he tried to remember if his mom had any troubles going through the menopause and realised, she probably went through the worst of it when he was at school.

Karen began proceedings by carefully describing her menopausal experience. She did indeed pass through it when Leigh was at school. Because he only visited for short times during those years, he never once noticed anything in his mom like what Emily was going through. Karen said the physical changes can have a devastating effect on mental health. She explained that her method was the opposite of the HRT approach. Of course it was. Her physical issues were very problematic. She had hot flushes all the time, her head banged, and she felt repulsion instead of attraction to his dad. However, she said she didn't want to compress or hide the symptoms of the transition. Instead, she wanted to accept the changes as essential and natural, and she focused on treating the mind instead of the body. It worked for her.

Karen described a scene to Leigh that he could've never imagined. Seven women in the grips of menopause, experiencing very difficult times, all sitting cross-legged on the floor in a converted school bus, preparing for a ritual. The magic mushroom tea was measured perfectly by an *old crone* hippy elder woman, and each woman was given a cup filled to the rim with a brownish elixir. They were asked to embrace the changes coursing throughout their physical bodies and told to drink as much tea as they could in ten minutes. When they finished, they all sat there for about half an hour before a heavyset woman, dressed in a Japanese-like robe, began laughing. She tried to suppress it, but she snorted, and everyone in the circle began to double over in hysterical laughter. Many of the women hadn't experienced uninhibited laughter for months or years up to that point. It was a scene of heaving bodies of all shapes, sizes and skin tones, sharing a superconscious experience.

As the psilocybin trip deepened, each woman began to self-examine her life at that moment, what she had been through, and what was possibly to come. It was a profoundly mind-altering experience that was personal to each but had an obvious common thread. *This is mother nature, release and accept.* When they came down from the trip, each one was changed in a special way. One woman was adamant about never doing anything like that again and wanted HRT straight away. That was her journey, Karen said. The rest of the women either had a few more trips to cope or used microdosing of psilocybin daily to help the mind and body work together better. His mom stressed that this was a path that had been proven to work for thousands of years before modern medicine.

Because Dr. Emily had spent so many hours in A&E with recreational drug patients, she was totally against those types of drugs. Leigh, on the other hand, was raised in a relaxed environment of cannabis, LSD, MDMA, nitrous oxide balloons, and just about any other recreational drug out there. He'd left that life behind when he married his doctor wife, however, it now seemed that the past might need to become the present to help shape the future. But how, he thought?

Dr. Emily's moods were off the charts, and both daughters were hardly ever home to avoid the drama. Leigh decided on a drastic manoeuvre.

"Hey Em, fancy playing a board game later? We haven't done that in ages." He asked. Emily looked into his hopeful eyes, tiredly, and said, "Sure, but after a glass of red."

"Brilliant! Hey, I don't know if you'd be interested or not, but I bought some special tea that might help with *the M word,*" Leigh hesitantly stated. "Would you like to try it before the Merlot?"

"Ah, jaysus Leigh, I've tried nearly everything I can think of," she said in response.

"Ok, but I have it from a very reliable source that it does

help some women sometimes," he countered. "Who's the source?" "My mom." Emily's eyebrows rose to a peak on her forehead. "Your mum!!? What have you told her? When did you talk to her? I don't feel good about you talking to her about me, Leigh," she said in a rather harsh tone.
"I spoke to her a few days ago. I only told her the truth, Em. We're not in a good place at the moment, and I asked if she had any ideas. You wouldn't believe the story she told me about herself. I decided to give it a shot, but you know you don't have to," Leigh finished.

Surprisingly, Dr. Emily softened her tone and posture. "I didn't mean to snap at you. I know you want to help. Thank you. I suppose I've nothing to lose, and I trust you. I'll try it," she said.

Dr. Emily was absolutely blown away by the tea. She knew he was trying to help, and he'd only ever been caring throughout the failed process of her HRT exploration. She knew he was well-educated in such areas, and his mum was very intelligent. In the third hour of her trip, she was crying and laughing at what it means to bring a child into this world. In hour four, she saw what she was going through and all the failed medical procedures that she had been so skilled at for other women, but which had not only failed, but had backfired on her. She realised her transitional process and understood why she hooked up with the man she did. She came down from her trip with no headache or itching, and she actually felt attracted to Leigh for the first time in ages. She needed an occasional cup of tea every now and again, but for the most part, the mushrooms were her answer.

Six days after her first experience, the irksome symptoms were making a comeback. Dr. Emily decided to FaceTime Karen and ask questions that only she could answer. The two wise women chatted for almost three hours. During that time, the separate worlds of artificial medicine and natural remedies found common ground. Each woman came away from that conversation with new knowledge in areas that were previously only superstition in their minds. Karen learned how HRT was a lifesaver to countless women, and Dr. Emily learned about natural healing and treatments that were once common thousands of years ago, before the pharmaceutical industry made them taboo. Karen suggested a few books for Dr. Emily to read to gain a deeper understanding of the science behind the remedies. She devoured the literature and expanded her arsenal of weapons against the menopause. She felt relieved and relaxed going forward, delighted she had found something that helped her.

Dr. Emily had a new outlook on what she now referred to as *natural plant medicine.* She lived by the credo that *everything happens for a reason.* She considered how poor her quality of life was and would have been if she'd never met or married Leigh. Most of the time, her conventional medical treatments helped her menopausal patients. On the very rare time it didn't, she had a magic ace up her sleeve for a different type of woman. Feckin Hippies, she thought with an internal chuckle.

The funeral was attended by only a few close friends and family. James was in deep shock and numb at his new reality. He was in a place where he wanted answers but also to be absolutely alone. A few of his mates looked him in the eyes and said they were there for him anytime, and they meant it. James couldn't bring himself to believe that only last week, he and his wife had a dinner date to try to rekindle the embers of their marriage. It was an okay date, but not great. Then, two days later, he came home to find she had taken a bottle of sleeping tablets and two bottles of wine. She was blue and cold to the touch, so he knew she must've done it just after he left for work that morning. The coroner officially ruled it an accidental overdose because it was a prescribed medication, Xanax. Jame's head was in a deep black hole of despair. He couldn't begin to imagine a life without his wife.

It was three o'clock in the morning. James was out on another long walk because of a sleepless night, trying to make sense of what had happened. He hadn't realised it had been years since things seemed normal in their marriage. As time is a master trickster, it only felt like weeks or months since things felt normal, but surely not years. That fact alone was a massive smack in his face, and James felt miserable about himself because he hadn't been a more attentive husband. He felt sure there was something he could have done to help. It was a thought much too late, and it consumed him. James hated himself and needed to find answers to change that feeling.

Their relationship began as any fairy tale might. The ensuing years were both rocky and lovely, as all marriages are. Intimacy was part of daily or weekly life. Dirty remarks and grabbing some sexy flesh were always welcomed for years and years. It seemed like life in the golden years would be lovely and intimate. However, a fairytale ending to a fairytale beginning was not on the cards. It was more like a horror story written by Stephen King.

James sat tucked under an overpass bridge again at 3 am, shivering in the cold and rain on a local road, and watched cars go by at that early hour. He wondered how many people inside those cages were having similar struggles. The petrol and diesel smell wafted up inside the bridge-tunnel. A boy racer and a Harley-Davidson went under the bridge. That made him feel better. Rebels were still out there, he thought to himself. He smiled an aching smile as he listened to the last sounds of the Harley in the distance. The smell of someone burning turf came through the tunnel from somewhere. James began to cry hard again.

He felt a more profound and deeper anguish at the prospect of having no companion to share the last stage of life with. He left his place under the bridge and went for a walk to reflect. The road he shuffled along got steep and narrow as he strolled. James took the footpaths with the least resistance and found himself at the entrance of the largest graveyard in the area. That felt like precisely the right place to be at that moment. He turned on his phone's torch and began to read the grave markers. The pattern was soon obvious: if a man passed away first, his partner usually lived much longer. If the woman passed first, the man passed in a few years at most, in many cases.

The anguish turned into despair as he realised this was not only because of the practical everyday things they shared, but also because the man had a deep longing to not be here without the being that stirred his soul. The graveyard became a frequent destination for walks many nights after midnight. Nobody knew he was even going there. It became his happy place in the days and nights of despair. The only word to describe his reality at that time was total and unequivocal *anguish*.

James had kept reasonably fit over the years to remain healthy and attractive to his wife. He was also very helpful around the house. The raw laws of nature look at this as trying to make yourself desirable to your mate. James considered all the unfit and unfriendly lads his age who were making no effort to be attractive. The catastrophic penny dropped. They didn't care about their appearance because it wouldn't matter if they were Hercules; their woman, like his wife, wouldn't have had any interest. He thought that if they had a spouse at that point, they must only be coexisting, which must be horrible.

It was another day at four o'clock in the morning, the anguish deeper than ever. Reflection and meditation offered no answers inside the graveyard, and the despair of existing without his wife became a living nightmare. The torment deepened, and depression set in hard. Reflecting on the very tragic passing of men in their forties and fifties who took their own lives made much more sense now. James would not consider that path for himself because of a deep belief that you have to come back and do it all over again if you press the reset button. Empathy for these lads and their families came pouring out, and the compulsion to do something to help became an overwhelming obsession. James needed to determine why so many marriages failed after twenty or more years together.

The next morning seemed brighter than the past days, and the oppressive fog cleared a tiny bit as he shuffled around the empty kitchen with his cup of coffee. The floor was mucky with graveyard dirt from the night before. James didn't care. His days consisted of trying to sort out the household affairs his wife had seemed to handle effortlessly over the years. James knew her phone passcode, and she had written all her computer passwords in her diary. He had total access to everything she was doing up to the last day of her life.

She was a member of two Facebook groups about the menopause, and she had also followed several people on Instagram who were involved with menopausal topics. James had no idea why she was into that subject. He felt self-loathing for this ignorance. The Instagram posts were terrible enough, but the Facebook posts on what the women were going through shocked him to the core. Each post he read was like a jigsaw puzzle piece with absolutely no place to fit. The symptoms varied remarkably, and desperation was evident in each heartbreaking post. He found himself thinking that he was surprised more women didn't choose to do what his wife had done. A tiny bit of research revealed that what his wife had done was quite common at her age. James felt he'd stumbled into an alternate reality the deeper he researched. Why wasn't anyone talking about this, he wondered?

James next went into his wife's e-mail account. Nearly all were work-related except for three. Those three were an exchange between his wife and the coordinator of a women's menopausal group in South County Dublin. His wife was reaching out for help from this group, and the woman said her group would most definitely help. His wife was due to attend a meeting the next day. They were all looking forward to meeting her, the email finished. This was crushing because it felt like she was still alive for an instant, and she would be attending the meeting. James was very tempted to turn up and tell his story, then learn more about what had happened to his wife, but he decided a phone call in advance would be the correct thing. The call was answered before the first full ring, and it wasn't at all what James expected.

James had been chastised and criticised by many people in his life, but the way the coordinator of that menopausal *help* group spoke to him on the phone had his ear still red, and he was furious. "What the fuck do you want now?" "Sorry?" James said. "I thought you were someone else, sorry, what can I help you with?" said the voice on the other end. James stammered, "I'd like to attend your next meeting about the menopause."

There was a grunt of disbelief, and her voice was still loud and angry. "That's not going to happen, you're a man and have no business in our meeting. Your presence would undermine the integrity of the group, and you'd make the women feel uncomfortable. Menopause is a woman's issue, so goodbye," the coordinator hissed as she abruptly hung up the phone.

James didn't get the chance even to say why he wanted to attend the meeting, or that his wife was dead. He was stunned numb and properly pissed off at the nasty exchange. He nearly rang her straight back to let her have an earful, but he chickened out.

James felt an intense yearning to learn about the *menopause beast* that took his wife away. He sat down at the computer and did some research. James emailed two other groups. All he wanted to do was attend the meetings and listen. James had learned from the phone call to the rude coordinator that he needed to tell his story first and then request attendance. He didn't want to be spoken to like that ever again. The two groups were sympathetic to his story but insisted that their groups were for menopausal women only. No men allowed, ever.

James was shocked. He'd never felt the emotion of discrimination in his life. He had been drinking when he read the replies. He was raging and vowed on the spot to begin a *men-only* menopause group and never let any women attend. He laughed out loud at the absurdity of what he'd just thought. Discrimination and drink can lead people to do outrageous things and beginning a group like that was either courageous or crazy.

James approached two of the three lads who looked him in the eyes at the funeral and explained what he was setting up. He knew both were going through difficulties in their marriages, and he suspected the reason, but none of them knew anything about the menopause. Now, James desperately yearned to change that. He set up a group called *Understand Menopause*. He then asked his mates to ask any other lads who might have trouble understanding their marriage difficulties to attend. James then went to work to find experts who could explain the menopause. He assumed it would be hard to find teachers, but he simply went to the website of the Dublin group, copied the email addresses of all of the presenters, and hired two.

The first official meeting of *Understand Menopause* was attended by him and two of his mates. The first of two speakers he had paid in advance arrived outside the house and was shocked to be met at the door by a man. She dressed in flowing dark red robes, and her spiked hair was dyed bright blue. She seemed to be wholly triggered at the thought of speaking to men. She flat-out refused to enter the house, then took out her phone and immediately refunded the money James had paid her. He was shocked, hurt, frustrated and angry.

The second speaker was due in an hour. James wasn't off to a great start. One of his mates made fun of him for trying to set the group up, and James had to admit it was a bad beginning. The lads took out their phones to pass the time, and James suggested texting friends, saying there was free beer at the meeting. That worked. Six more men were on their way. James scampered to the off-licence to buy beer. All nine lads were happily drinking when the second speaker arrived. She certainly wasn't what anyone was expecting. She was cool.

She drove a Toyota Hilux king cab truck with a topper over the truck bed, and looked like she could line out for any men's rugby team in the country. Her hair was styled into a high bun, and she had a short, buzzed undercut around her head. Her gait was like that of a lumberjack, and she dressed in red and black plaid, so she also looked the part as well. With no other information, she gave her name, Sara, then took in the scene before her. Nine middle-aged men were getting drunk and apparently wanted to learn about the menopause. Sara could never have imagined teaching in a room like that. She grabbed a beer, cracked it open, and suggested they begin the meeting.

"Menopause is probably the worst thing that can happen to a loving man and possibly one of the best things that can ever happen to a woman," she said with her beer raised high above her head.

Sara hadn't taken a drink yet but knew how to read a room. She said, "Women need their space and room to blossom after the years of fertility have passed." She continued, "Those years are sometimes the hardest years many women would ever experience."

Sara then tipped the beer bottle into her mouth and drank it all in one go. This woman was a pure force of Nature, and as the evening rolled on, she had four more beers. She explained the menopause in a simplistic way that dumb drunk lads could understand. When the evening ended, they all walked home, and Sara declined an invitation for a spare bed in James's house. Instead, she opened the back of her Hilux and climbed in. It was kitted out as a sleeping truck. She was some woman for one woman, he thought. Initially, the meeting went off the rails, but Sara reaffirmed his drive for this mission.

The next meeting was set up a month in advance, and James had a ginger mate who had been pestering him to break his rule that no women were allowed. The ginger lad said, "James, my wife is changing, and we both see it happening. She doesn't want to see doctors just yet. We don't know enough to understand what's happening, but if my wife could listen to Sara just once, she could grasp the process."

James hadn't yet booked any speakers for the next meeting, which was a worry. He hadn't considered having Sara return. But why the hell not? She knew what she was getting when she arrived, so there'd be no surprises. One quick phone call to the lumberjack lady, with the ginger lad standing next to him, and she was booked as the only speaker for the next meeting. Sara insisted on free beer again.

And James gave the ginger lad permission to bring his missus, of course.

The anguish James experienced each day was still present, but the mission he was now on to help other men, and now couples, understand the menopause was helping to lessen the pain slightly. It still consumed every fibre of his being, but he felt better now that he was doing something to help. James continued to frequently take walks in the graveyard in the early hours of the morning, and the bone-crushing version of his anguish was there, but less somehow. He often thought about that first meeting and how it had already changed how nine lads understood the opposite sex, going through the menopause, better than most of the human population. He also found himself thinking of Sara, and the total mystery that she was in such an interesting and unique package.

The evening of the second meeting arrived. Eight of the nine friends were there again, and only three said they were there for the beer as they laughed. Three wives were present, and their energy definitely changed the room's dynamic. James now saw how a man in a woman's group would do the same. He noticed the lads weren't as loud or messing around as they had been last time. However, the last time, everyone was pretty well lubricated when Sara arrived. This time, when she entered the house, everyone was sober. That was another major factor in the different atmosphere. This felt more like an actual meeting and less like storytelling at the local pub.

Sara came directly to James, hugged him, and congratulated him on a better-looking crowd than last time. She knew his story and greatly admired what he was doing. Sara grabbed a beer, and everyone sat in a mishmash of chairs in a semicircle. She picked up a chair, turned it around backwards, threw her leg over, and straddled it. She opened her beer with a keychain yoke, toasted the room, and once again knocked it back in one drink. Sara cleared her throat and tried unsuccessfully to muffle a beer burp. Everyone laughed, and she began to teach not only about the menopause but also about her personal journey.

Sara wasn't a lumberjack after all. She was, in fact, a nurse in a women-only clinic, in her fifth year of the menopause, and didn't have an easy beginning. The room was sombre, and she was very good at reading it. Sara spoke quietly and thoughtfully this time. Last time, she was like a storytelling Viking. This time, Sara was like a university professor. She had chameleon-like properties, James thought to himself.

He realised that Sara was a very, very good speaker. She made eye contact with the women when she discussed symptoms that might make a lad squirm and with the men when she made points about loss of libido.

She then dropped a bombshell, "I know everyone here probably assumes that I'm a lesbian by my manners and how I look, but I was married to a man for twenty-two years," she said with a laugh. "And yes, the menopause was a major factor in my divorce. I was sick of the man I had married and decided this time in life is mine and mine alone. I dress like this to keep the men away," she concluded.

Everyone laughed as if it were a stand-up comedy show as Sara reached for another beer. Toward the end, the meeting took on a question-and-answer format, and the women had a few good ones. The nurse answered every question with compassion and wisdom.

When everyone was finished, she thanked them for attending and asked them to tell their friends about the group.

The meeting ended, and Sara and James stood beside her truck as she rolled and lit a cigarette. He knew she would say no, but he offered the spare room to her again. Sara took a drag, blew out the smoke, and said to him, "I had a great time with your group tonight. It was undoubtedly the best meeting I've ever taught at." Sara then turned to walk into the gaff, looked over her shoulder and asked, "Where's that spare room then?"

The two of them settled into the lounge room and began to chat. Sara said, "Last week I was at a meeting and mentioned what you were doing with your group. Some of the women, after the meeting, asked if I thought you'd let them attend. So, I'm now asking on their behalf. And I want to come back next month if you don't mind. I have more information to share, and I won't take no for an answer," she finished.

James found himself agreeing to everything Sara suggested. He said, "You are the expert here; I'll do anything you want. As you know, I started this group from a drunken temper tantrum. I'm delighted you're staying; it'll be the first night I won't be in an empty house in months. Thanks," James concluded.

There would be no anguished graveyard walk for James that night. The next morning, Sara had helped herself to tea and toast before he woke. He liked how she made herself at home in his home. He'd slept better that night than any other night since the funeral. They went over a plan for the next meeting. "I suggest you find a hall because I'm going to speak to other groups next week, and I'm going to invite women to invite their husbands along to the meeting. You know, James, you are a bloody genius to develop this idea to help men and women," she said. They said their goodbyes, and James looked forward to seeing Sara next month.

Sara was true to her word. The next meeting was at the local GAA hall, and there were many unfamiliar faces. And, at Sara's request, no free beer. This one felt like a proper meeting. Sara dressed in her usual garb but was most definitely in professor mode. She stood at the door and greeted the women she had invited from the other groups; many of them had brought their partners with them. James scanned the crowd and couldn't believe that his drunken hissy fit, because of a rude coordinator had made him establish this group in just four short months. He thought he felt a smile somewhere deep inside himself. James squashed it as quickly as he felt it. He didn't deserve to smile at all. He should've been a better husband.

Sara returned the following month with a surprise guest speaker. Sara asked for a round of applause as she introduced a woman responsible for setting up a menopausal group in Dublin. The guest looked around the room nervously before beginning to speak. James recoiled in his chair when she started talking because the speaker's voice was the same one that chastised him all those months ago. He had to fight the urge to stand up and kick her out! James was furious, and the red mist descended. He glanced over with eyes full of rage at Sara. She smiled wickedly, gave him a wink and put her finger to her lips in the *shush* gesture. James trusted Sara, so he calmed down a little. He was so grateful for everything Sara was doing, but was seething that the bad-mannered coordinator was there.

The speaker began, "Thank you all for coming to learn about such an important time in women's lives. My name is

Mandy, and this is the first time I've ever addressed any group with men in attendance. I must admit, it's the only time I've been nervous in years," she confessed.

Mandy then asked about the whereabouts of the courageous man who had established the group. James was so stunned that he simply raised his hand as if he were back in school. Mandy looked him in the eyes from the front of the room, put her hand on her heart, and offered the sincerest public apology anyone had ever heard. Mandy complimented him on his inclusive group and admitted that it was good when both men and women were interested in the menopause.

Mandy said, "In the small social media circles on the topic, this group is being heralded as a major advancement in learning about this subject." She started a round of applause. James was floored. Of course, he knew nothing about this, as men aren't allowed in menopausal social media groups.

Mandy spoke for over an hour and was incredibly easy to listen to when she got rolling. James was impressed by her charisma and, reluctantly, noted that she was also very attractive. James hated to admit this because he had made Mandy into a sort of *she demon* in his head with horns and fangs and shrivelled up pasty white skin. Instead, she looked to be in her late fifties and was in fantastic shape. Mandy had a deep tan and long brown hair with a striking grey streak that began at her left temple. James had to admit she was one of the most captivating women he had ever seen. He laughed inside at the strange twist of fate that had led to that moment. It dawned on him then that he had just laughed inside for the first time in ages. And the woman he had directed his *grief anger* at was responsible for it.

Sara didn't speak at that meeting because Mandy was so brilliant. It was by far the best meeting they had had to date. Mandy approached him when the crowd thinned out and offered her hand. "James, I had no right to speak to you the way I did, but I do have an explanation," Mandy confessed.

Sara walked by and interjected, "And James would love to hear it in his lounge room with a few drinks."

"That's a great idea, and I need to thank you, Mandy, for speaking to me like you did. We wouldn't be here now if you hadn't been so bloody rude," James said with a chuckle.

On the walk to his house, Sara blurted, "My truck is my bed, and James has a very nice spare room for you, Mandy, so let's have some drinks and chat for a while." James was a bit shocked, but he was now used to Sara's straightforward style, so he said, "That sounds like a good plan. What do you think, Mandy?"

"Are you sure, James? I don't want to intrude, but I'd like that if it's not too much trouble," Mandy replied.

The talk was small between James and Mandy while Sara smoked a rollie outside. When Sara returned, she predictably waltzed into his kitchen and grabbed four beers. She opened one for each of them and raised hers in a toast to *three warriors who are trying to help humanity*. She drank it in one go again. James was impressed every time she did that. Mandy and he each took a swallow as Sara sat down and opened the fourth beer, then took a swig after a massive belch. That broke the ice as they all roared with laughter.

Sara blurted again, "Mandy, why don't you explain to James why you spoke to him like a sailor on the phone the way you did." Mandy took another swallow of beer and began, "Not two minutes had passed when you'd rang, since I'd hung up on my ex. We got into a massive argument. He's a master gas lighter and was on form that day. He knew exactly how to push my triggers. When you called about possibly attending my group, I thought you were him ringing me back. I was ready to unload with both barrels. Unfortunately, James, you got shot instead. I'm so sorry," she apologised yet again. "That makes sense," James said. "I'm sorry for your troubles, and apology one hundred per cent accepted."

Any tension that may have been present immediately evaporated. James and Sara knew each other's life story, and Sara knew Mandy's, so Mandy cleared her throat to fill James in on how she began the group she so adamantly denied him access to. It turned out to be a mission for her as well. Mandy began, "I tried hard to hold my marriage together, but the menopause broke my body and spirit. My ex is the type of man who is grumpy, demeaning and condescending if he's not getting sex regularly. I tried to go through the motions for a while, but in the end, I just couldn't do it anymore. He began seeing other women and didn't even try to hide it. He would be texting his girlfriends in front of me just to put me down. That was the final straw. I hated him for this."

James stared intently into Mandy's eyes and recognised a familiar look, *anguish.* He hated her ex too and experienced a rush of empathy. Only a few short hours ago, he wanted to stand up and kick this woman out of his meeting, and now he wanted to stand up and give her a massive hug. He didn't. They all chatted for another hour. Sara said goodnight, then went to her truck. James showed Mandy to her room, and he went to his. As he lay in his bed, he allowed the anguish to return. It was powerful, and he broke down and cried. He missed his wife, and he felt that if he had been more attentive, she would still be alive. Then his thoughts drifted to the bizarre fact that the woman his wife was going to ask for help from was sleeping in the next room. And if his wife were still alive, he would never have met Sara or Mandy. James knew his group was helping people because he got emails almost daily thanking him and Sara. He really liked Sara. She was possibly the easiest person to be around that he'd ever met. The anguish lessened by one degree. He then thought about Mandy, and the anguish lessened one degree more. He didn't know what he thought about her; he just thought about her.

Sara's truck was gone when James and Mandy woke the next morning. It was a typically cloudy and blustery day, with showers on and off. The night before, there wasn't any discussion about how Mandy would get home. James assumed Sara would give her a lift home since she brought her down the night before. There was no way Mandy was going to take public transportation in the bad weather, so James knew it was up to him to give her a lift home. This didn't upset him even slightly; in fact, he was looking forward to it. They had two cups of coffee and a piece of toast before getting into his car for the hour-long journey to her house. They got along very well. James found that ironic, considering their first interaction.

Mandy invited James into her two-bedroom cottage outside a small village in Kildare. He thought she lived in Dublin because that was where she held her group meetings. He'd pictured the nasty coordinator as a snobby South Dublin hag. He was dead wrong. Mandy explained she used the building there because it was offered to her for free, and it's a more densely populated area. Her cottage was small but very nice and cosy. A wood-burning stove in the lounge room and the dark Liscannor tiles in the kitchen gave the cottage a very old-world feel. There was a computer on the kitchen table and only two chairs, so it took up very little space. It looked like a comfortable living space, and he said it to her. “Your house is lovely, Mandy, it’s like a postcard or on the set of The Quiet Man,” James said.

Mandy smiled when he complimented her home. “It was a gift to myself when the large house my ex-husband and I jointly owned was sold after the divorce,” she explained. Pointing to the table, she continued, “It was at that table that I took your phone call and ripped your head off.”

They laughed at how absurd that sounded now. James mentioned he had to get home as the wind and rain were picking up. They said their goodbyes, and he left for home. James chose to go through the stunningly beautiful Wicklow Gap. It was spectacular even in the wind and rain. As he admired the otherworldly beauty, he let the anguish flood him again. He braced himself for the avalanche of despair he’d become so accustomed to. The anguish punched him in the chest, and it hurt like hell, but it didn’t consume every cell of his being like it always had since the funeral. James pulled the car over at a scenic lay-by and prepared for the tears. The tears always followed quickly after the anguish hit. He waited, but in the end, only wiped away two tears. That was another first. He should've nearly been doubled over, sobbing uncontrollably, but he didn’t feel the flood coming. James remembered that the last time he let the anguish in, which didn’t nearly kill him, was last night while thinking about Sara and Mandy. He didn’t know what was happening, but thought he might feel almost good for the first time in months.

Mandy's group meeting remained a *no-man's zone,* as some women would never attend or seek help if men were present. James understood that now. He saw firsthand how the opposite sex changed the energy in his group. His meetings went from what was essentially informative but glorified pub sessions to solemn and educational meetings. His group was consistently well-attended by both couples and singles every month.

The night they all stayed at James's house; Sara stated that he was a leader in the menopausal movement. He never took her seriously; he felt like a big impostor because he knew nothing back then. It dawned on him that he had listened to so many sessions and stories and responded to countless emails that he must be one of the most informed men on the menopause in the country. His group was one of the only inclusive groups, so he was gaining fame in a tiny community. He accepted the role of a leader in helping couples find understanding and, hopefully, solutions to the menopause monster that took his wife.

James stayed in touch with Mandy at least once a week and found himself inventing reasons to contact her. It would always be related to the menopause, and she would always reply quickly. He was considering the idea of maybe asking her out for a coffee to talk about anything at all when his phone rang. "Hello, James. How are you?" Mandy asked. "I'm grand, Mandy, to what do I owe the pleasure of this phone call?" James asked smiling. He couldn't believe he was about to text her when she rang him. "I was wondering if you would consider attending our group meeting and telling your story next week. Most of the women are familiar with you now, and when I said I knew you, they were asking me questions I couldn't answer. I said I'd ask you to come

personally, so here I am, asking," Mandy explained. James was in stunned silence for a minute. Mandy said 'hello?' three times before James regained his composure.
"Sorry, Mandy," James said. "I don't know what I expected you to say, but it certainly wasn't asking me to attend your group. I'd be happy to do it on one condition: you return the favour in two weeks," he finished.

Mandy immediately agreed. Both were delighted when the conversation ended, not only because they would have a special guest speaker, but also because they would see each other again, two weeks in a row.

James spent the next few days in a mad panic, accompanied by a rather anxious yet soothing comfort. He had to speak to a group of women interested in the menopause, but whenever he finished, he looked forward to time with Mandy. His mental state was all over the place. He desperately missed his wife, but it had now been well over a year since the funeral, and he was painfully lonely. James knew he had genuine feelings towards Sara because he'd never met a human like her but had to admit that he fancied Mandy. James felt horrible self-loathing for thinking of anyone other than his departed wife. He took another walk to the graveyard at 2.00 in the morning and invited the anguish to punish him as hard as possible. It didn't come. He didn't cry. He felt something so foreign that he wasn't sure he was feeling it correctly. It was peace.

James went out and bought a new suit for her meeting. He usually dressed more like the lumberjack, Sara, but he had feelings that he hadn't felt in well over a year. James eagerly looked forward to doing whatever he needed to do so he could spend time with Mandy again. He knew he looked good in nice clothes, but he hadn't made any effort for years, which hurt him again. Maybe she'd still be here if he dressed a bit better back then. James knew that sounded crazy, but he'd become accustomed to blaming himself as much as possible for her death: himself and the menopause.

James was introduced to a group of about thirty women. The women were told via email that he would be presenting, and many women were attending just to hear his story. They knew part of it from the email, but many wanted to hear exactly what happened, and they wanted to meet a man who cared so deeply about a female topic. James asked Mandy about Sara and was told she wouldn't be there. He found himself disappointed. Mandy introduced James, and he spoke with clarity, wisdom, passion and authority. Some of the women cried during the hour-long speech. And he cried a little himself when he described the scene he walked into the morning when he found his wife cold in their bed.

When he finished, there were many excellent questions; to his surprise, he could answer most of them. He was swift to admit if he couldn't answer one. He never tried to fabricate an answer. He would just say he didn't know.

James stood in the car park after the meeting ended, talking to Mandy. He wasn't looking forward to the drive home and was just about to ask her out for an evening coffee. "James, you were great, and it's late, would you like to stay at my cottage for the night? My couch pulls out into a bed. I don't know how comfortable it is, but it would be better than the long drive home," Mandy said. "After all, I stayed at your gaff, you should stay at mine." Pretending to be calm and casual, James said, "I'll stay over tonight if you stay at my house again after you present to my group next week."
"Deal," Mandy said, and reached out for a handshake. James took her hand, pulled her closer, and hugged her lightly.

When they parted, each was smiling as much as the other.

They sat at Mandy's small kitchen table, shared a bottle of wine and had some cheese and crackers with homemade relish. James was happier at that moment than at any time in the past year by a long shot. He helped her pull out and set up the couch. They said their goodnights and planned breakfast at the local hotel the following day. He lay down and looked up at the ceiling of the cottage. James opened up to the anguish. Sadness descended. Loneliness descended. Guilt descended. But there was no anguish. He smiled at his peace and looked forward to seeing Mandy the next morning.

Following their meeting the next week, they took a long walk and discussed anything that came to mind. They both knew there were developing feelings for each other. Sara wasn't at his meeting again. It was as if she had just dropped off the radar. When he mentioned it, Mandy said she had been in touch and Sara was dating again, so she wasn't as involved in speaking as she used to be. James immediately felt a small wave of jealousy. He laughed inside at that, then thought that whoever was dating that nurse was one hell of a lucky person. For a short time, James had to admit that, in the past, he was hopeful of being that person. But as he looked at Mandy walking beside him, she smiled, and he desperately wanted to hold her hand. With no words spoken, she reached out her hand and took his in hers, and they slowly walked back to his house for the best weekend of his new life. He had fulfilled his mission, and his anguish just about vanished.

BEYOND MARRIAGE COUNSELLING

Maggie and JP had attended four marriage counselling sessions together. Maggie was also attending a Reiki practitioner for energy healing separately. She was willing to try anything. It was early days in the attempt to save their marriage, but so far, so good. Maggie's moods were calmer as she tried to live in the present moment. The best thing she had done was turn off the news for good and changed her approach to social media, which helped massively. The area of their relationship that was still quite dysfunctional was between the sheets. They had sex the night JP returned from the hotel and again four days later. But that was it. And it didn't feel like *making love*; it felt forced on her part.

There wasn't much conversation at the Reiki sessions. However, before the last one, Maggie made a feeble stab at humour and asked the healer, "Is there any chance you could *Reiki some horny* into me?" They both laughed, but when the session ended, the healer asked, "How serious are you about your sex life?" "I'm dead serious," Maggie said. "I love my husband to bits, but I have a hard time having *romantic notions*, if you know what I mean," Maggie finished with a wry smile.

The healer nodded understandingly and handed Maggie a blood-red card with only one word, written in thick black letters, covering the entire front: TANTRA. The healer said, "The website on the back of the card has all the information for the couples' retreats. Mind you, they're not everyone's cup of tea." She winked as she said it.

Maggie had sat in her car outside the healer's office and had a quick glance at the Tantra website. Her initial impression was a stunned shock, and she quickly assumed that this particular cup of tea wouldn't be to their liking. However, as she drove home, the idea of a retreat like this ignited a spark of passion that she hadn't felt in a long time. The website explained there would be group sessions with all couples present and private, one-on-one sessions between partners. It listed meditation, breathing exercises, eye gazing, and deep hugging. It also mentioned becoming comfortable with the body you have.

JP had just returned from the golf course and was freshly showered when Maggie entered the front door. He smelled terrific to her. They greeted each other with the customary kiss. Maggie asked, "How was the golf?" JP replied, "It was better than usual, thanks. How was the Reiki session?" Maggie smiled slightly at that and said, "I'll tell you about it over a glass of wine in a bit."

Later that evening, they sat beside each other with the laptop open on JP's knees. Maggie poured their second glass of red wine as JP finished reading the preliminary description of the Tantra retreat. Maggie had read all of it in her car, so she left him to it. He put the laptop on the coffee table, looked at Maggie, raised his eyebrows and asked, "Are you serious?" "I think so," Maggie tentatively replied. They didn't do things like this. They were a non-practising catholic couple. People like them didn't do these things. Not so long ago, it would have been akin to worshipping Satan.
"Let me show you something; it's a photo that interested me," she said. Maggie clicked on a tab she had looked at earlier. It showed a couple in a tiny room, tastefully naked, locked in a seated embrace. They had straddled each other's

legs and had their legs wrapped around the backside of their partner. Their crotches were close but not touching, and they leaned forward so that the weight of one would support the other. They were pressed chest to chest with their arms encircling one another. Their heads were resting on their partner's shoulders. It was beautiful to Maggie, and this image lit her spark in the healer's car park. JP stared at the picture and clicked a few more. There were more nude couples in various positions of seated and lying meditation, and many more photos of couples locked in various non-sexual embraces. These pictures made Maggie feel slightly aroused, and JP had to shift his position slightly on the couch. He was quickly becoming erect. She noticed his predicament and giggled. With the wine's giddiness, Maggie teased, "The Tantra appears to be already working."

JP laughed, dropped his hand below to shift a bit more, and then reached for his wallet. They booked a three-day retreat scheduled two weeks later. They finished their glass of wine and went to the bedroom for a very rare, passionate lovemaking session—the first heartfelt session in ages.

The retreat location was on the grounds of an old estate that had converted an outbuilding specifically for various groups to conduct retreats of different sizes on a multitude of topics. The stables had been expertly fitted out, so each tiny stall was private from the adjoining ones. The outside looked like a typical long-stone building with fifteen sturdy doors securing the privacy of the couples who would attend. The doors were stunning to Maggie. They were a kaleidoscope of colours. Each door was a different colour, with a top and bottom half. There were no others of the same colour. That's how you knew your room, not by number but by colour. Maggie and JP were given the *green door* stable.

This is where they would not only perform some of the one-on-one rituals with each other but also sleep on a double bed ingeniously chained to the far wall. They would let it down each evening with a rope through a pulley attached to the front of the frame. It was a small space, but it was beautifully decorated with various glossy Eastern deities in tasteful frames on the walls and even one that was affixed to the underside of their bed. There were a few single narrow shelves that held incense burners and candles. The floor was warm due to the underfloor heating installed during the conversion. It was tiny, but it was amazing.

The *break-the-ice* meeting was held in the early afternoon when all six couples had arrived. They were each handed a schedule of events. Some activities were group, and some were private, with just the couple and the facilitator present. It was the first time it had crossed their minds that another person might be present when they were starkers in their stable. JP wanted to say something. He instantly noticed that Maggie had just now copped on. She looked as mortified as he felt. JP reached for Maggie's hand, and she quickly grabbed it. They both squeezed harder than usual, looked into each other's eyes, smiled and raised their eyebrows simultaneously. They nearly burst into laughter. The forbidden type of laughter that overcomes you as a young one in Sunday church services. However, they instead winked at each other, took a couple of breaths, composed themselves, and directed their gaze at the tall, tan and toned facilitator standing at the front of the yoga hall. The hall was the only modern structure on the grounds. It was built of scented cedar and was spacious. It could hold thirty students, so the twelve of them, plus the teachers, made the space look massive. The wood stove in the front was burning heavenly-smelling birch logs, and the tapestries hanging from each of the four walls were stunning works of Far Eastern spiritual art.

The only two pieces of non-Eastern work were prints by Georgia O'Keeffe, which hung on either side of the wood stove. They were flowers, of course, but the teacher called them yonis. He made clear the significance of the sacred property, art and retreat.

The tanned teacher explained, "This retreat has blessings emanating from the very ground beneath our feet. It is built on a bedrock of quartz. The energy here is immense. The artwork around you and decorating your rooms is intended to engage you, inspire you, and bring you pleasure to look at. The retreat you've all chosen has been successful for every couple who has ever attended it. Some were successful in remaining a couple, some were successful in terminating the contract that had been fulfilled, and some simply returned to rejuvenate their relationship." He nodded to a couple on the middle mats at the far side of the hall.

Neither Maggie nor JP knew what the other was thinking, but they were feeling the same thing at that moment. They each desperately wanted to be in the first group the teacher had mentioned. Another mutual squeeze of their hands followed. The students were informed on this first day that they would soon have a vegetarian meal and an extended meditation session before heading to their respective stable stalls. The food was delicious, the meditation was awkward since neither of them had done it before, and the sleep was fitful on a strange bed in a strange place with a few strange days ahead.

The morning routine consisted of communal ablutions, which were awkward for all the couples. There were two compostable loos and three showers for them to figure out how to share in their varying stages of undress. Each stable stall had a night bucket for a wee. The serious business needed to be completed in an uncomfortable, compostable toilet, compacted by multiple layers of strangers' poo and sawdust. This was disconcerting to a very private lad who played GAA, was named after a Pope, and was raised catholic. JP shat and covered his layer with a scoop of sawdust. All this was new but stepping outside his comfort zone amidst new couples trying to improve their relationships, like they were, was unexpectedly invigorating. Maggie returned after her sawdust poop, and they shared a laugh.

"Did you flush properly?" JP jokingly asked. Maggie laughed and said, "I did one generously sprinkled scoop over the vegetarian mess I made." They both erupted in a fit of laughter at that. Having secured their bed to the far wall, they slowly strolled to the yoga hall, unsure of what to expect next. They were both excited, and this served to strengthen their bond.

JP and Maggie were the first couple in the dimly lit, yet beautiful, hall. With the pick of any of the pairs of mats before them, they selected a couple of mats at the far back left corner of the room. They intuitively knew each wanted to see what was happening before them. They suddenly noticed the completely motionless beautiful couple facing them on either side of the wood stove at the front of the room. They were sitting cross-legged and were wrapped in Indian homespun cotton shawls that hid everything except their heads, which were silver covered in cascading locks of long hair. Their age would be hard to guess, maybe early sixties. They appeared to be statues.

The last couple came in just as the bells sounded for meditation to begin. This couple was forced to the front, and it was evident that the anxious woman was trying her best to make her partner happy to be there. He wasn't. His body posture was rigid and uncomfortable, and the pair was tense. Maggie gave a slight nudge to JP and glanced in their direction. JP gave a slight nod back, knowing what she would say. It was like an entire conversation had taken place between them. They looked at each other and smiled.

The last chime of the bell faded, and the facilitators at the front of the room raised their arms simultaneously. Their shawls fell off their tanned torsos while vibrational tones from hidden speakers began to saturate the hall. The vibrational tones seemed to flow into their ears and flood their entire body. The theatrics were very good, thought JP. The incense and stove's birch wood made for a very heady olfactory experience. The hall was only candle-lit, so it took a short while before everyone present realised, they were looking at two teachers who were naked from the waist up. They obviously spent a fair amount of time without their shirts on in the sun's magnificent rays. His chest was taut and muscular, with broad, rounded shoulders. He had a hooped ring piercing each nipple. Her chest was beautifully adorned with small breasts that were only slightly sagging. Her areolas were large, and her nipples were pert and pointed upwards because of the slight chill in the hall. They didn't look sexual; they looked beautiful. They opened their arms in unison and began chanting a low, vibrational "OOOMMMMmmmm…" All the couples took the hint and started to join in the chanting, except for the last ones to arrive. He was now gawking at the female facilitator, and his partner fiercely elbowed him to get him to stop.

The chanting ended after fifteen minutes, and the male facilitator slowly stood up without warning. It was as if he had a rope under his shoulders and simply went from seated to standing with no effort. As he stood, the rest of his shawl fell to the floor. He stood before them naked as the day he was born. He'd apparently had more than just his shirt off in the sun. There were no tan lines anywhere. He calmly began to speak to the group as if he were wearing an Armani suit and giving a TED Talk instead of being totally naked except for the hoops in his nipples. He began by explaining that Tantra was the path of the heart. It is about the sensual as opposed to the sexual. It is divine love, not human love. He asked everyone to stand and close their eyes. The female facilitator and another couple dropped off their robes. This couple were the veterans who would help out during the next few days. All were naked.

When everyone stood with their eyes closed, the female facilitator began to speak softly, just loud enough for Maggie and JP in the back to hear.

She said, "The human body is only a suit of meat that allows the soul to be a functional vessel for an instant. It is a lifetime for us but a blip in universal reality."

She instructed, "Everyone should try to feel comfortable in the body you have, as it is now. If you want to make changes to your physical appearance, create a plan and work toward it. But love your body every step along the way. It possesses a portal to sensual pleasure and awakening opportunities. The yoga hall will always be at the current temperature. From now on, clothing is optional within these walls and on the sacred land. Being comfortable with your body is hastened by the lack of concern from others who are unclothed. It soon becomes the natural way to feel. In one minute, we'll begin an energy-boosting exercise. The less clothing, the better."

She instructed them to keep their eyes closed and invited the couples to whatever state of dress or undress they felt comfortable with. There was a rustling of clothes for a short time and then silence. She invited everyone to open their eyes and prepare to dance.

Maggie and JP quickly adjusted to the dim lights and noticed that only they and the couple in front hadn't removed a stitch of gear. The veteran couple, or *angels*, were nude, as was a younger man with an older woman. She had her bottoms off but kept her jumper on. The other pairs were mainly down to their knickers. One younger woman had her yoga top still on, like the jumper the older lady wore. Maggie quickly glanced at her husband, then at the uptight couple at the front, and back at JP in a virtual nanosecond. She crossed her arms on either side of the bottom hem of her jumper and whooshed it over her head just before JP had unzipped his GAA tracksuit top, and they theatrically gave the garments a swirl by the sleeves and threw them down at each other's feet. They had no idea what had come over them, but each knew they didn't want to be lumped in with the tense couple in the front row. JP broke first. He nearly choked as he tried to suppress the laughter erupting from below his comfort zone's crust. He burst! Maggie exploded and let out a whoop from God only knows where.

The hall erupted in gales of laughter. Vibrant Indian music burst into life, blaring from the hidden speakers. The facilitators and the angel couple began to dance in half-rhythm and half fits of convulsions. The other students initially started to mimic the motions, but they soon developed their own expression of awakening energy. JP had only danced in GAA settings, so to be topless amidst a group of strangers had him outside his comfort zone by miles.

Maggie had on her sports bra and yoga pants and was bouncing and twirling with her head back, eyes closed, and her arms outstretched. JP was sucked into the moment of weirdness, and without a second thought, on a very frantic tempo that was getting faster and faster, he hooked his thumbs into the waistline of his underwear and tracksuit bottoms and bent over, then quickly stepped out of them. He was naked!!! This was the first time it wasn't family or teammates. He was naked in front of strangers, and he loved it. His bleach-white body glowed like an LED headlamp. He laughed from his heart and then tapped Maggie on her hand as it twirled by. She looked at his beautiful body, and without stopping her twirling, she removed her top. She stopped for an instant to pull down and step out of her bottoms. Immediately, she began twirling again, and JP giggled as he did a spasmodic two-step on his mat.

The Indian *jigs and reels* continued for fifteen minutes. All the couples were naked at the end, except for the nervous couple. The older woman had removed her jumper to reveal a stunning chest tattoo where her breasts had been before a double mastectomy. The younger woman had removed her yoga top to reveal a large birthmark between her breasts that looked like a jar of hot Nutella had spilt there, and tiny hairs grew from the edges. Nobody cared a rat's arse what anyone else looked like at that moment. Nearly everyone was aware that something special was happening. They were all full of energy. Even the anxious couple were down to their underwear. It was craic like Maggie and JP had never envisaged. Everyone was instructed to lie down on their backs and let their sweat trickle down the awakened flesh of their bodies onto their mats and breathe deeply in through their noses and out of their mouths for several minutes.

The corpse pose meditation and cool-down period lasted ten minutes, and a deep bell signalled the end of the morning session for the day. There would be a meal in two hours, and as the two silver-haired beings left the hall, everyone seemed to snap back to reality. The sweat had cooled on their bodies as they lay on the floor, but they weren't cold. The anxious couple was first up. In a fairly comical way, they hurriedly dressed like their parents had phoned, and said they'd be home in five minutes. The older lady put her jumper back on straight away, as did the younger one with the birthmark.

Almost everyone had put on at least some clothing.

Maggie and JP were still lying on their backs when the nervous couple and two other pairs left the hall. Neither felt like moving a muscle, but they began to reluctantly roll over and find their clothing. Nobody was speaking. Everyone seemed a bit stunned. JP motioned with his head for Maggie to look out the large window at the tanned facilitators. They were strolling along a path to the main house at a snail's pace. They were hand in hand and stunningly naked. Maggie looked up into JP's eyes and just nodded. They both gathered their clothes in a ball and tucked them under their arms. They grabbed each other's hands and walked nude to their green door stall. It wasn't a slow stroll, but it was invigorating to be the only couple to leave the hall in their birthday suits.

Maggie closed the stall door behind them and turned to hug JP passionately. The love he felt for her made him bring himself so far outside his normal boundaries, filling her heart with bliss. They embraced in a full-body hug, their bellies and chests pressed together, with their heads resting on each other's shoulders. No words were spoken. The expression of pure love emanated from them both and permeated the tiny room. Maggie slowly released the embrace and reached for the rope to lower their bed. They had two hours before they had to eat. They made sensual, slow, love like spiritual beings for an hour before emerging from their green door to walk to the shower stalls. They were still nude.

Following the meal, everyone was to meet again at the yoga hall. The anxious couple was the first to arrive this time, sitting in the same spot where Maggie and JP had earlier. Maggie wondered what JP's reaction would be. He nodded to them and walked up to the front, where they had sat. Maggie thought it was a classy move on his part. Before taking a seat, JP surprised her by unzipping his top, removing it, folding it, and placing it on the floor next to the wall. He did the same with his bottoms and jocks. He was naked again. Maggie wasn't one to be left out and copied his actions, then sat to join him on the mat. Both crossed their legs as best they could, sat up straight and closed their eyes to meditate and wait for the others to arrive.

After a short while and some rustling behind them, a bell sounded to bring attention to the facilitators at the front. They were beautifully nude once again. Maggie snuck a cheeky quick glance around the room and noticed every single person was unclothed. The anxious couple seemed to have calmed, and they, too, were now nude. Everyone was instructed to lie on their left side to aid the digestion of the meal they'd just eaten. They all stayed in that position for twenty minutes. There were sounds of people sleeping all around the room.

When the bell sounded again, they sat up and were instructed in vigorous breath exercises. They were told to inhale deeply and quickly through their noses, hold their breath for a count of three, and then exhale explosively through their mouth in two powerful puffs. The hall immediately sounded like a storm was blowing a gale inside the four cedar walls. All the huffing and puffing nearly had Maggie and JP in the giggles again, but the energy of the space seemed more serious and sacred than the first time they were there in the morning. After only three minutes, which felt like ten, they were instructed to sit in total silence, focusing their mental attention on a point between their eyebrows and simply observing the breath moving in and out of their bodies. They did this for fifteen minutes.

The bell chimed. The sacred woman facilitator nodded to the *angel* couple. They rose and wove their way around people to the front of the class. A plush sheepskin rug was placed on the floor before the wood stove. The male sat down with his legs straight and his arms planted on the rug behind him to support his weight. His partner walked up to him, so her torso aligned with his face. She parted her legs and sat down on his lap as though they were going to have seated sex, facing each other. They didn't. As she settled, she pressed her chest into his, and he, in turn, leaned forward, put his arms around her body and pulled her close. This was the couple JP and Maggie had seen in the website image. They looked so beautiful, locked in this passionate and sensual embrace. They barely moved, and in a short while, their breathing seemed to synchronise. They seemed to breathe as one unit. It was beautiful to look at, lasting five minutes, which flew by as the class watched. The female facilitator congratulated the class on their comfort zone to be natural. She said it rarely happens so quickly, and they would do another round of wild and crazy dancing to get the energy moving. They would then lie in the corpse pose briefly before going to their stalls to replicate the demonstration the *angels* had done. A facilitator would knock on their coloured door and enter to assist the couples in achieving the best results. They were instructed to do their best independently until the teacher arrived.

Indian music started prematurely, and everyone just popped up and started their version of dancing. The facilitators and angels added coughing, hacking and laughing into the mix. The students followed suit, and soon, everyone thrashed around, making guttural noises as if they had a slug stuck in their throats, and laughed at the spectacle. It was a free-for-all compared to the morning session. Couples bounced, laughed, twirled and coughed away from their partners. Everyone was dancing with everyone else. It was like a teenage disco, except everyone was stone sober and bare-arse naked. JP was dancing next to the older woman with the chest tattoo, and Maggie was dancing with the partner of the woman who had a Nutella-like birthmark. They pranced, jigged, twirled around, and soon danced with the young, formerly anxious couple. Eye contact was minimal, but the energy pulsating was palpable. The young couple was soaking up and basking in the energy that Maggie and JP were letting loose. It was a heady experience.

When the corpse pose ended, the awkwardness around nudity was minimal this time. Everyone rose from their mats and filed out of the hall carrying their clothing to their respective coloured doors. JP opened the door for Maggie, and they quietly entered the stall and closed the green door behind them. Maggie retrieved the rolled-up sheepskin and placed it on the warm floor of the tiny stall. It was strange that neither had spoken yet. It felt like words would spoil the moment, so they continued in silence. JP sat down, and Maggie mimicked the demonstration, straddling him. It should have been erotic. It wasn't. It was sensual and as beautiful as the *angel* couple earlier. They pressed their chests together and lovingly wrapped their arms around one another. They gently laid their heads on each other's shoulders, and their breathing slowed. They were warm and perfectly comfortable. Their breathing began to synchronise, and before long, they were one being composed of two halves breathing together. The gentle knock on the door didn't startle them; they didn't move a muscle or even open their eyes. They heard the door open and close as someone entered the room. They felt someone near them for an instant and could hear the shuffle of bare feet. And the next instant, the door opened and closed again. Whoever it was only stayed long enough to see if they were doing the practice correctly. They were. They felt amazing.

The next day was a carbon copy of the previous, except everyone was now totally comfortable. It was amazing how it happened so quickly. The five couples there for help were now almost as comfortable being nude as the angel helpers in the yoga hall. Even the anxious couple seemed chilled now. They were going to last as a couple a wee bit longer, at least. Maggie realised that she and JP were possibly the stars of the class. A lad named after a Pope immersed in the GAA wouldn't be a typical Tantra workshop student. Maggie loved him deeply. She felt the same longings and stirrings that she had when they first began to get intimate before they married. She knew his longings had never diminished. Maggie's fire was re-ignited.

The weeks quickly turned into months, and Maggie found herself taking online classes in cooking and writing. JP received a promotion at work. His hours were very unpredictable, so Maggie was spending more time alone than she was used to. She particularly loved writing and found it came naturally to her. The first writing she focused on was simple journaling. She had a diary as a young girl and had forgotten how much she loved jotting down a few lines about her day. This small act of self-reflection led her to begin the act of considering the necessary steps to rebuild some of the bridges she had burned in the past. It would be no easy process, but she was determined to salvage anything she could with her friends, but most importantly, her sister.

Maggie began to write fictional short stories about self-empowered women. As she did this, she felt a spark ignite a flame within herself. She was able to weave a narrative effortlessly. The creative process awoke feelings long buried by time and life circumstances. The central focus would always be the mental health of her characters and the steps they took to achieve well-being. She wrote a story about a hormonally unbalanced woman who had a massive fight with her sister at a women's protest, and they hadn't spoken since. When she finished, she emailed it to her sister. Thankfully, it worked. Maggie and her sister reconciled within a week after Maggie sent her email.

One down, several to go, Maggie thought to herself. She repeated the process with each of her former close friends and was able to rebuild the bridges that she had thought were beyond repair. Her social circle was expanding within just a few months, and Maggie enjoyed the freedom that JP's irregular hours afforded her. She admitted to herself that the new position at work didn't suit her husband. The stress of the promotion was causing JP sleepless nights and had him in foul humour most days. Maggie found it difficult to even talk to him as he wasn't allowed to divulge anything about what he was investigating in any case. The more delicate she was with him, the more aggressive he became. Maggie began to plan the hours of her days to be away from home when he was there. It progressively accelerated day by day and week by week until Maggie felt compelled to confront the situation.

Maggie had fixed a meal to be ready for the time he said he would be home. He was very late. She kept it warm in the oven for over two hours, and when he finally arrived, he went straight to the shower, muttering that he'd had fish and chips in his car earlier. Maggie wanted to blow her top, but didn't because she remembered that she had, in the past, acted the same way that he was now acting. Maggie was full of compassion and empathy and realised that this must have been the way he felt about her when he produced the divorce papers and suggested marriage counselling. She knew it was time to turn the tables on him to get things back on track. Maggie got a few sheets of blank paper and a blue crayon with an A4 envelope. She wrote on the top of the page, DIVORCE PAPERS. She then made squiggling lines, like small rippling waves, on the remainder of the page. She repeated the squiggles on the other pages and then put a line in place for two signatures at the bottom. Then, like a school note to a friend, she drew two small boxes.

One said *divorce,* the other, *marriage counselling,* followed by the phrase in parentheses, *put an X in the box.*

She heard him turn the shower off and hurriedly shoved the schoolgirl pages into the envelope, leaving it on the kitchen table as she scurried into the lounge room. JP went from their bedroom into the kitchen to grab a beer and noticed the package. He sat at the table and opened it. As he looked at the contents, he actually burst out laughing. Maggie's heart filled with hope and joy. A fresh and clean JP joined Maggie in the lounge room, and he only said "touché". Maggie laughed, and the angst of the past few weeks seemed to dissipate like the water on a footpath following a short rain shower in a hot summer sun. They laughed at the ploy, and JP agreed to be more agreeable in the future. They had the best night together in weeks. Maggie was still blissfully asleep when JP woke up early for an emergency call-out the next morning.

Maggie woke up an hour later to do some writing. There was a knock on the front door, and she looked at her watch. It was exactly 11:11. Usually a good omen, she thought. Maggie closed her laptop on the story she was writing for a local short story contest. She was in a flow and was irritated by the interruption but put on a good face to greet whoever was there.

She opened the door to JP's supervisor. He was looking down at his feet with his cap in his hands. When he raised his gaze to meet hers, it was clear this was not a good omen. His eyes were bloodshot, and his face was ashen. He cleared his throat but still spoke with a soft raspy voice. He informed her that JP had been shot in the back during a raid of a well-known drug den and is fighting for his life in St. Vincent's Hospital.

The Spanish holiday was predictably platonic. Ryan kept a playful mood around their two kids, but inside, he was broken. He had a successful business, beautiful kids, a stunning-looking wife, and a house that she remodelled to her taste, which he hated but was getting used to. He decided to try to make the best of a bad situation. His parents had left him their business and home when they were killed in a motorbike accident on their Spanish holiday when he was only twenty-four. He loved their rustic style and hadn't planned on changing it. However, when his wife, Fiona, began *the change*, she took it upon herself to completely gut the house when he was on a business trip for their shop. It went from a rustic cottage feel to Ikea in under a week. He took up running to escape. It worked.

Ryan's marathon training kept him extremely fit, but it also kept him away from his wife for long periods of time. It was painful for him to be around her because he still loved her and fancied her rotten. Ryan didn't like what she had done to their house and how she treated him, but he still wanted to be with her. It was during a training run on that holiday when it occurred to him that he might know a way to spend time with his beloved and not have to communicate too much. Ryan had entered a meditative state at around mile seven and let his mind wander to Fiona. He thought about how they met when she needed a tyre changed and how she naturally seemed to fit into his life like a key into a lock. Fiona was a great mother to their kids and knew how to invest money. She had made them more money than he had ever dreamed of. Fiona mentioned at home while packing for the trip that she hoped the resort had a gym because she wanted to get fitter. He had a plan.

Dinner that evening was in a modest restaurant that the kids loved. They served pasta and pizza. It was filled with noisy families on their holliers. Ryan took out his phone after they had ordered and opened up an album of his running photos. He scrolled to the very beginning when he was unfit. He wasn't fat back then, but he was overweight and could only run 200 metres on his first go. He showed the kids what he looked like. and they laughed hysterically. They said he looked so much younger now than he did then. Ryan chanced it and asked Fiona if she wanted to have a look. She reached across the red and white chequered tablecloth and took his phone. She put her hand to her mouth and smiled at his appearance. Fiona looked up at him and back down at the photo on the screen.

"The kids are right; you look so much better now," she complimented, her surprise evident in her voice. "Thanks. Running has changed my life," Ryan replied. He then played his hand.

"Would you like to begin training with me? You said you wanted to get fitter," he said. "We won't chat much while we train." Fiona shocked him by saying, "Hmmmm, I'll have to think about it. It sure worked for you." Ryan smiled inside.

The following day, Ryan woke first and went for coffee, as usual. He was only gone fifteen minutes, but when he returned to their room, the kids were dressed for swimming, and Fiona was togged out head to toe in running gear. "The kids are going to swimming lessons. They will be gone for an hour. Will that give us time for a run?" Fiona asked.

"It will be more than enough time for your first run," Ryan

replied. Fiona passed the one-kilometre mark before stopping. "You're a natural," Ryan said to her as they strode along the path back. Fiona turned her bright red face to look at him, saying, "Running is pure hell." Ryan laughed from his belly and told her, "It will be like that for a few weeks, then it will be the opposite of hell."

Fiona said nothing else on the walk back, but Ryan didn't care. He was happy to be doing something with her. They showered separately, dressed, and collected the kids for breakfast. She dressed in the ensuite as usual, but didn't close the door completely. Ryan desperately wanted to see his wife's naked body, but he had learned his lesson and stayed well away from that side of the room. When she emerged, he thought she looked absolutely stunning. He said nothing. While they ate breakfast, she was more talkative than usual. Fiona asked the kids about the lessons and asked Ryan if they could do another run in the morning. He smiled at her and simply nodded. Could his plan be working?

They ran together again the following day, but this time, Fiona asked him several questions about running on the kilometre walk back. Ryan happily answered each one. He had asked the same questions of his coaches when he began, so he sounded like he knew what he was talking about. He actually did. They chatted more like a trainer and an athlete than a husband and a wife, but he was grateful for any little crumb she would toss his way.

It was the last day of the holiday, and Ryan was curious if they would continue to train together when they returned to Cork. They did. They ran together each morning. They picked a route that would be a short loop for Fiona. He would say farewell at their drive and then do a serious training run on his own. His thoughts would always be about

Fiona and how they were beginning to get along better. It wasn't his imagination. She was in better overall form around the house during the day and sleeping better than she had in ages. It had taken almost a year working with her doctor, but her HRT seemed to be balanced now, and her fitness was steadily improving. Fiona began reading books on diet, nutrition and the menopause. She began attending a healer and a therapist for her mental well-being. Fiona dove into her self-care as ferociously as she dove into financial investing. This combination had her in the best form she'd been in for years. Ryan was hopeful.

The first time they ran together in a race was the Tramore Valley Park run. They were at the start line at 9.25 am for a 9.30 start. Fiona was understandably nervous and bouncing up and down on her toes. She had run a full 5 km just the previous week without stopping. Ryan suggested it was time for her to do a race if she felt like it. She was ready. They had only trained on concrete surfaces, so she was slightly worried about the gravel path aspect of parts of the course. He assured her she had nothing to worry about. They completed the 5,000 meters in just over forty minutes, and she was both ecstatic and exhausted in equal measure as she crossed the finishing line. They had a coach-student relationship the entire time they had been running, but she hugged him after catching her breath and thanked him. Fiona did that like a wife, not a student. Ryan was ecstatic inside.

The fifth park run saw them dip below the thirty-minute mark for the first time, and Ryan suggested they double the distance and do a race where you actually paid to enter and received a shirt and medal upon finishing.

Fiona eagerly agreed. She had the running bug, and he was over the moon that they spent so much time together training.

Fiona's fitness had improved dramatically, and they were now chatting while on training runs. The chat was always related to running, the kids, the business, or their investments. It was never about their relationship, but it was progress, nonetheless, in his eyes. Fiona was as chatty now as she had been on their first date. Her mood around the house, especially in front of the kids, was always cordial and sometimes playful, but rarely with him. That was changing. She began to ask if he wanted a cup of tea occasionally, like she used to, and he always accepted, even if he didn't particularly want one.

They had run only three 10k races before signing up for a half marathon in Waterford. It was called the Viking Half, and Fiona aimed to finish in under two hours. This was a big ask because her best 10k time was fifty-seven minutes, and she had to maintain that pace for twice as long. Ryan ran beside her for the first 10k and then shot off alone. He wanted her to use the two-hour pacers to experience running with a group of strangers of similar fitness.

One of the pacers began chatting with Fiona and complimented her on her running form and fitness level. The pacer asked what club she was with because she was obviously well-coached. When she said her husband was her coach, the pacer was impressed and told her so. Fiona felt a surprising wave of pride for Ryan wash over her, and that put a renewed pep in her stride.

The finishing line was inside a proper stadium, and the final 400 metres was around an athletics track. Ryan was shouting support for her on the last 200-metre stretch.

Hearing his voice had the effect of spurring her to kick hard. She passed both the pacers with 100 metres left and finished the 13.1 miles in 1:58:59. Fiona was over the moon and threw herself into Ryan's open arms. He gave her a congratulatory hug, then added an extra little squeeze for his own sake. She reciprocated the last hug, much to his surprise.

The October Bank Holiday Monday was crisp and clear with no rain in the forecast. They had trained hard the past few months for this very day. In Ryan's opinion, the Dublin City Marathon was one of the best in the world. Ryan had run loads of marathons, so Fiona trusted his judgement She was still two different personalities. She was his attentive and motivated student during training but was still only a friend around the house. She was a much friendlier friend than she had been before the running started, but their relationship remained strictly platonic. The course in Dublin was challenging but very enjoyable. The supportive cheering from the crowds was present from the beginning all the way to the end. Autumn leaves in the mature neighbourhoods littered the road, and the ones still clinging to the long limbs made a beautiful tapestry for the eyes to feast on while the body pounded out the miles.

The 200-metre-long blue carpet to the finishing line was a welcome sight ahead. Fiona kicked on harder, and like the half marathon, Ryan was on the other side of the line waiting for her. The embrace was incredible. She was in tears of joy and relief. A photographer snapped their photo and took their names.

They slowly collected their belongings from the bag drop area and headed to the car. Fiona was full of chat for the first hour on the way home but then became absorbed in her phone. Ryan didn't know what she was doing, but she was in charge of the investments, and he totally trusted her. As they pulled into the driveway, her phone rang. When she answered, the conversation was brief.

Fiona agreed with the caller for 5:00 pm and hung up. She looked at Ryan and said, "Fancy a look at an investment property with me tomorrow evening?"

"Yup, I'm happy to do anything with you," Ryan replied, hoping not to let his desperation show.

The next day, they stopped for a coffee at a local shop, and their picture appeared on the front pages of all the papers. They were the new promotional photos for the following year's Dublin City Marathon. The couple looked at each other in utter disbelief. They bought a copy of each one and laughed like teenagers as they put them in the car. It was late afternoon, and they would be late for the appointment if they didn't get a move on.

The drive to the property took them only ten miles outside Cork City, almost thirteen miles from their house. The rural road was narrow with a mossy robin in the middle and had no markings. The tall, mature trees on either side of the road created a tunnel-like sensation as they drove under them.

Fiona turned the car into a narrow laneway that curved around to a circular drive, in front of the most beautiful, thatched cottage Ryan had ever seen. The whitewashing was pristine, and the green trim around the windows made it look like a John Hinde postcard Ryan thought to himself. He was shocked that she would consider an investment property like this. Fiona had modern taste, and this cottage wasn't her style. However, this was right up his late parents' alley. Ryan loved the outside, but the inside was even more spectacular. The massive stove in the lounge room was the centrepiece of the cottage. There were only three other rooms and a loo.

The lounge room had two high-backed chairs facing the stove and a small, round-topped table between them. The internal walls were bare stone, and the windows had wooden shutters inside that locked tightly closed to keep the weather out and the heat in. They were painted a vibrant red. Ryan loved the colour scheme. The kitchen had a modern gas cooker and a small, square table in the middle of the room, surrounded by four chairs. Fiona put the kettle on and took two cups out of a well-stocked press. Another press revealed a box of tea, and when she opened the small refrigerator, there was a pint of fresh milk there. He was in love with the property but was completely confused. Why was it stocked with tea fixings? Why was it painted in his favourite colours? Why was she interested in a cottage when she worked so hard not to have it in their home? Fiona sat at the table and handed him his cup of tea and a set of keys.

Fiona had purchased the cottage for him immediately after they completed the Viking Half Marathon in Waterford. She was so grateful for his training and for being there for her without expectations or pressure as she worked hard to manage the menopause. She wanted to do something special. Ryan was speechless. Her turning their formerly rustic house into a modern home had started him running away in the first place. Well, to be honest, the changes in the house and herself had him running.

Fiona had changed even more since they began running together. Ryan tried to stop looking at her as his lover ages ago. It only caused him sorrow. He loved their time training together, but life in the family home wasn't like a married couple. It was more like two friends who were minding kids they loved with their heart and soul. Fiona looked into his eyes and reached her hands across the table. He blinked twice, looking at them before reaching across, clasping them gently, and squeezing them harder. A tear ran down his left cheek, and she raised her right hand to wipe it away.

Fiona sat back in her chair, cleared her throat, and sat up straight. She began by taking a deep breath in through her nose and out through her mouth, as she did when trying to get her breathing correct on a run. "Ryan, I'm very sorry. I had absolutely no control over my feelings or actions. I was all over the place," Fiona stated. "Thank you for sticking with me. I know it wasn't easy. I love you more now than ever."

Ryan didn't know what to say. He began to tear up properly. Fiona excused herself to use the bathroom and struck a match in the well-prepared stove on the way. The flames burst into life, and as she turned, her figure was illuminated in the bright orange glow of the fire. She was beautiful.

The toilet flushed, and Fiona emerged. Instead of returning to the table, Fiona made the short trip from the bathroom to the only bedroom in the cottage and closed the door. Ryan was puzzled, to say the least. She returned to the table with a bottle of red wine and two glasses. Fiona was wearing a nightgown that wasn't suitable for the outside temperature. She motioned him to the stove and sat in a high-backed chair facing it. Ryan was in total disbelief. Standing slowly, not to disturb the mirage he was experiencing, he walked carefully over to the tandem chair while she filled the two wine glasses. The cup of tea forgotten. Fiona handed one to him as he sat down. They clinked glasses without a word. He was used to not talking. They stared into the glass stove door and silently sipped as the flames danced on the logs.

Again, without speaking, Fiona stood and extended her left hand towards him. Ryan grasped it and stood immediately. She gently tugged him in the direction of the cottage bedroom. He couldn't believe what was happening. He stopped in his tracks and asked her if she was sure? Fiona gave him a long-lost wicked smile and a wink, and then her face softened. She looked at him pleadingly. She assured him. Ryan was convinced. He was on cloud nine. He had his lover back and an authentic cottage in homage to his parents. It was worth the wait, the trouble, and the turmoil. He was no longer a broken man.

A HAPPY ENDING!

Their sailboat was coming into the harbour after a day around the coast of Dublin. It was a bright, brilliant day; the sea smelled fresh and briny. The sun shimmered with glowing, golden rays, reflecting the tips of waves like a disco ball. Sunglasses were essential. It was perfect. The heat was welcome, as it's usually cold in St. George's Strait. The occasional sea spray as the boat dipped was welcome on John's face. He looked over at his wife of twenty-seven years, Helen, and saw the same beauty now as he had all those years ago when they were introduced by a mutual couple, Neill and Mary. It's sad, John thought to himself; their friends were divorced, and they hardly ever saw either one any longer. John now understood that their friend's marriage fell apart when Mary was going through the menopause. John didn't know that then. Nobody understood what was going on in those days. He'd hardly even heard that word, as nobody ever seemed to talk about it. He smiled at Helen; she smiled back. John counted himself a fortunate man.

Helen and John had two grown children. Both kids had moved away from Ireland in 2010 when the recession crippled the country. Young people had no choice. They had to emigrate if they wanted to work. Helen almost instantly changed with their departure. She was always sad and went into what they thought was commonly called *empty-nest syndrome*. They had many friends whose kids grew up and emigrated, so it must be normal. They assumed this phase would pass eventually. It didn't.

Helen hid the pain behind her eyes from everyone. Well, almost everyone. John could see the sparkle in her eyes had dimmed, and she had become withdrawn at home. Helen stayed in bed in the mornings longer than ever, after seeming not to have slept at all the night before. She used to be a very early riser, and most mornings, she would have a walk before her first cup of coffee, no matter the weather. Helen was always a tiny bundle of energy. That was when the kids were home. She rarely seemed to have the energy to get through a day, let alone go for a walk.

John watched in silent anguish as Helen drifted further and further away from him. She was like a boat with no rudder. She was stunning. Helen was five feet five and filled with gunpowder. Her long hair was always pulled into a bun on the back of her head. She was the envy of other women her age. In bygone days her stride while walking was just short of jogging. She dressed the part then as well. Track suit and a rain jacket on inclement days. Yoga tights and a tight top on better days. Those times were over.

John began to stay later at work to minimise the time spent at home watching the woman of his dreams slowly go deeper and deeper into the darkness of the empty nest syndrome. He had always kept himself in good shape. John was a six-foot-tall former rugby player with a driven work ethic. He was hoping this situation was temporary. However, it did have certain advantages. This later working circumstance saw him increase their income noticeably, but there was very little joy in having fiscal freedom without the love of his life to share it with. John was finally financially secure but had no way to purchase a cure for the crippling depression that had gripped his wife.

John was trying to help and suggested a possible visit to the doctor. "Helen, you haven't been yourself since the kids left.

Do you think a visit to the GP might be in order?" John asked innocently. This question backfired. Helen recoiled as if he had struck her. She was a strong-willed, strong-minded and very independent woman who had always been the rock of the family. Helen exclaimed, "I certainly don't need a doctor; I simply need some more time alone."

She was born into a generation that didn't see strength in asking for help. Instead, it was a sign of weakness, and there were no obstacles that couldn't be *managed*.

Helen's *time alone* extended from four months to eight months, then ultimately to a full year. John's business was flying like a kite, but his marriage was sinking like the Titanic. He felt completely out of control with no options. He knew he needed to get their children home, at least for a visit. Thankfully, the increased income he'd been amassing provided the opportunity to surprise his wife. John thought an abrupt change in her circumstances might have a profound impact on Helen. He was letting hope creep in, feeling grateful.

John bought two tickets for their kids. The plan was put in motion to surprise Helen three days before Christmas. He had watched several YouTube videos of surprise homecomings, which were very popular in Ireland because many children had had to leave over the years. He felt hope inside and was excited to be the mastermind of what would surely break the grip of depression that was choking the very spirit out of his wife. Hopefulness was a welcome visitor at this point in his life. The long-awaited day arrived. "I'm heading to the office to finish up a few things before the long break," John yelled upstairs to Helen.
John was always at the office these days, so this wasn't even slightly suspicious. His reunion with their kids at the arrivals

hall at Dublin airport was very emotional. He knew in his heart that this would make everything better instantly. John hugged his kids and began to cry with joy, but mostly relief. His tears surprised his children because he hadn't even cried when they left separately over a year ago. The oldest asked, "You alright, Da?" "I sure am now," he said, hugging them again.

The trip home was full of stories of work and life overseas; however, John barely heard a word they said. He was trying to figure out how to explain what the past year at home had been like. He decided to stay quiet as this was, hopefully, going to be like hitting the restart button on Helen's life when they walked into the house again.

Helen had Face Timed the kids many times in the past year. She was her former, happy-go-lucky self during those chats, but the contact had become less frequent with the time difference and the amount of time she was spending alone. This was going to be a great Christmas. It had to be better than last year. That was the first Christmas with the kids away, which triggered her downward spiral. This was a rewind. It was a brilliant plan. John had high hopes it would work. They pulled into the driveway and beeped the horn until Helen appeared at the door. The meeting was incredible. Her look of shock and confusion was quickly followed by howls of joyous bawling, hugs, and kisses all around.

"Ahhhh Jaaaysys," Helen sobbed as she wiped tears with the back of her hand. "I can't believe you're really here. I've missed you both so very much. I love you rotten," she cried, taking them both into her arms again.

The reunion rivalled everything that any YouTube video had ever shown. Helen even threw her arms around

John and gave him a massive hug and kiss. The action was the first meaningful physical contact of any kind in months. John was hopeful for some actual intimacy and romance again. He felt he was a very thoughtful and romantic partner. She'd always brought out the best in him, and he loved to please her.

The kids were home for two weeks. John was one hundred per cent correct. Everything was back to normal, and it was like the past year was just a foggy, lousy dream that allowed him to make the money needed to make this magical moment happen. Helen was in flying form, floating around the house, full of energy. They all took a few walks as a family over the break, and Helen was the leader of the pack.

During those two weeks, Helen and John held hands and cuddled. They even made love a few times. She was so happy to have them home. He felt like a magician for being able to manifest this, and he was living with the person he remembered. On the last night of their visit, the couple who had introduced them to each other, Neill and Mary, came over to say goodbye to the kids. There was a very noticeable tension between their friends. Everyone tried to ignore it, but there was no denying that something was seriously causing friction.

It was time for the kids to return to their overseas homes. The two siblings hugged everyone, lingering in Helen's embrace as long as they could, then walked out to their taxi for the airport, luggage in tow. Helen stood at the front door with tears streaming down her face, watching the taxi until it was out of sight. She then returned to the tension-filled lounge room.

The wine flowed between the couples. As the evening wore on, Neill and Mary grew colder and colder toward each other. They had mini arguments about everything. It seemed to be Neill pushing Mary all evening, but both gave as good as the other in the end. One spat about the garden needing Neill's attention prompted John to interject. "Hey," John said to the group. "How about we all get away from this gloomy weather for a while, you know, take a holiday like."

Neill agreed immediately but added a massive twist to the plan. "Sounds good. Us lads will go away together, and you two women can plan something to do on your own. It'll do us all a world of good."

John was stunned, but Mary didn't miss a beat. "That's the best idea you've had in ages, *hun*," she sarcastically said as she looked at her husband, then rolled her eyes to Helen.

It was settled. The following week, Mary decided to book a retreat for her and Helen, and Neill booked a golfing holiday for the lads in Spain. John and Helen had very little input. They would all leave in two weeks and return on the same day. The two holidays couldn't have been more different.

The Women

Instead of leaving the country, Mary had booked a retreat in an out-of-the-way location in County Wicklow. The first afternoon, when the women arrived, Helen noticed that there were only women, which seemed to be of a particular demographic.

"Mary, I don't see any men anywhere," Helen said. "There had better not be any; it's a women's only retreat," Mary replied. "And everyone seems to be around our age," Helen continued. "Of course," Mary said, "they would have to be. Helen was confused but left it at that.

The retreat location was idyllic. Helen hadn't asked any questions about the retreat that Mary had booked. Helen felt she needed to be away from her husband again now that her kids were gone, and she knew Mary wasn't in a good place. Helen felt she was going to enter the same depression again now that her house was cavernous, lacking in life, and empty. She couldn't do anything to stop it, but she was here for Mary.

They carried their bags to the two-person hut they would be sharing. Helen casually glanced at the schedule of topics to be covered for the next few days that was left on the bedside table. She was shocked and embarrassed at the same time to even be reading it. This was a retreat for women with any interest in the menopause on any level. Helen wasn't interested in that topic and was frantically trying to think of what to say to get out of there as quickly as possible. She thought it was going to be a cucumber slices on the eyelids and pedicures retreat, but one session the next day focused on *reclaiming your vagina*, and another was *channel your energy back to you.* She felt like she got off on the wrong platform at the station and wanted to get back on the train and go anywhere but there.

"Ummmmm, Mary, what exactly is this retreat?" Helen nervously asked. "It's to learn about what we're going through," Mary casually replied. "My marriage is in the bin, and I've noticed you're not the same Helen you used to be, so I thought we could use some factual information."
Helen was flummoxed at this response and realised that there was no leaving. The property was in an isolated setting, surrounded by mountains and forests. The sea was

even visible from specific points. It was the perfect place to escape to if you needed to escape, because there was no escape from there. She felt silly for not asking Mary for details before agreeing to attend. She knew that her friend's marriage was on the verge of collapse. Helen was compelled to help personally. She believed her marriage was good for the most part, except that she just missed her kids in the gaff.

They organised the room and themselves, then made their way to the main chalet. An area in the back of the packed room suited them. The first forty-five-minute talk was given by a mature woman who was about six feet tall when standing. However, when she folded herself into a seated position, she looked like she had collapsed into a suitcase. Her limbs were very long and somewhat large, but they were incredibly limber. The talk was about living in the present moment, familiar to someone who had lived for over five decades. Helen wondered if the speaker had children who had left home for money and to make a living. She felt resentful that someone would encourage forgetting the past.

The older woman didn't forget the past. The class was scheduled for sixty minutes. Following the lecture, a bell rang, and incense began to permeate the structure. Hidden speakers in the room's corners seemed to give off comforting vibrational tones. Helen was taken aback by the meditation exercise suggestions.

"If you are single or separated, think of every time you self-pleasured in the past year and why you did it. If you are married or have a partner, think of all the sex and intimacy you've had the past year, as well as the self-pleasuring times and again, why? If there is a void compared to the past, ask yourself why. This class is about remembering pleasure and acknowledging any lack of it that may have snuck away. Spend the next fifteen minutes looking inside yourself and ask silent, yet powerful, questions. Vegetarian food will be ready when you finish," directed the teacher.

The speaker wasn't suggesting that we forget the past but instead focused on a particular aspect of it. Helen had no idea what to do next. She didn't know anything about vegetarian food, and she certainly didn't want to sit on an uncomfortable cushion for the next fifteen minutes. She closed her eyes and tried to endure the time until lunch. Helen was there to help Mary out of the seemingly dire situation that led to this desperate holiday. Helen's breath calmed, and she went silent inside for the first time in ages. She felt, nothing. She was quiet, at peace for the first time in as long as she could remember. Helen only ever had energy for everyone else in the family, and at this moment, there was no family. There was only herself, and it was...terrifying.

Helen immediately remembered the glorious Christmas they all shared. There was sex and pleasure. She felt she didn't need this retreat. She was only there to support Mary because Christmas was a special time in her memory. Then, her memory slowly shifted to the previous Christmas. Helen recoiled inside as she remembered it had been at least that long ago since the last meaningful sex of any type. And she hadn't engaged in any self-pleasuring urges, she realised. Helen felt like another person watching the past year unfold. The kids moved away, and she went into a turtle shell of sorts. She had disappeared in any way, shape or form to her husband and everyone else. This realisation rocked Helen to her very soul.

She had never meditated before, and her worried mind wondered if she was doing it right. Wasn't meditation supposed to be peaceful? Helen was feeling anxious, the opposite of what she expected. Instinctively, she inhaled deeply through her nose and let it out from her mouth, and her thoughts calmed somewhat. She made the decision there and then to give this retreat her full attention. It had been less than ten minutes, and already she had made some profound self-revelations. Helen surrendered to her mind and let it drift to scan her body. She started with her feet and legs. They were tense, so she consciously relaxed them. She relaxed her stomach, chest, shoulders, neck and arms. Helen then subconsciously asked herself how she felt. Her body's reply was instantaneous. Helen was tired.

She had entirely forgotten the past year of being uncomfortable in her skin. She realised that her body hadn't slept soundly since her kids left the house, no matter how long she spent in bed. She would get very hot, then comfortable, then cold in the space of just a few minutes. The meditation was working. Helen began to understand she had changed drastically in the space of a year. She allowed herself to become completely immersed in the practice. All thoughts of Mary were gone entirely. This retreat was an eye-opener in many ways. Helen had no idea she was lost and had no words to explain the past year. She realised the symptoms had been creeping up on her for a while, but she was always so busy running the household that she didn't give them any merit.

The next few days were an epiphany as Helen realised she was in the menopause and that her life needed attention. Mary was attending different classes, as there were many on offer, and she chose the *separation-type* courses that focused on detachment and rebuilding. This worried Helen a bit, but she was now focused solely on herself and trying to make sense of what had happened over the past year. She went there initially to help her friend out, and now realised they were both there for different reasons.

The incense and vibrational tones of each class on the retreat were always potent, and Helen allowed herself to accept each class and lesson as what she simply must do. Each teacher seemed to agree that most women would never have to resort to manufactured chemicals to flourish in the autumn of their lives. Any discomfort within the body can be naturally overcome by what is provided in nature, as the menopause is a natural process. She listened intently and committed to this pathway as it felt right.

Diets and herbal remedies, as well as gardening and sparking a possible lesbian relationship, were all suggested by the teachers between the now-delicious vegetarian meals. Helen discovered a sisterhood that she had never even known existed. This was a chance for herself to reclaim her vagina and energy and all the rest of what she learned.

The drive back from the retreat was quiet. Each woman was contemplating what they had experienced. Both were equally driven to do what they felt was right in their heart. When Mary stood at her front door, Helen told Mary she was eternally grateful and knew what actions she must take. Mary smiled a sad smile and knew what she had to do, too. They hugged like they had never hugged before. They both knew one would try to save a marriage while the other was already dead.

The Lads

The lads arrived three hours early at Dublin airport for their quick flight to Spain. John was excited to go golfing with his mate and chat about their marriages. It was evident that Neill was having difficulties, and John hadn't mentioned his troubles to anyone yet. Neill was eager to hit the airport lounge for a few quick pints before they headed to the gate. John wasn't a big drinker, but what the hell? It was a lads' holiday after all. He was determined to have a deep chat with Neill, so if it took a few drinks to loosen the tongue, then a few pints of the black stuff would do nicely.

The second pint went down smoothly, and then John wiped the foam from his lip and cleared his throat. "So, how's things with yer missus? It was a little tense at Christmas. Is it all good now?" He asked.

Neill nearly spat out his beer. "If you don't mind, I don't want to hear a single word about Mary while we are away. She is the last thing I want to even think about for the next few days," he added.

Neill ordered a third pint, but John declined. "I'd have to piss every ten minutes if I had another," he said. Neill laughed, but John was crushed. If he couldn't even mention the wives, this would be a long few days. John initially thought this was the reason for the trip, but he now began to understand that this wasn't the case.

John began to feel uneasy as they made their way to their gate. Neill was ogling and commenting on every woman who caught his eye. Some of the comments were way too far. Three pints didn't excuse some of the things he said he would *do* to some of the unsuspecting women in his line of fire. Since it was only the first few hours of the holiday, John decided to say nothing and let the Guinness filter through his mate, but he had a bad feeling this was a big mistake as they made their way to the cramped seats on the Ryanair flight.

The lads arrived at the hotel/golf resort by bus, and Neill immediately went to the bar to order another drink and insisted John had one as well. They weren't golfing on the first day, so John decided to just go along with what his friend wanted to do. Neill brought the drinks to the table and pointed to two dark-haired women sitting together at the far end of the bar. The bartender delivered two drinks to them, and the women both smiled, waving at the lads. John was beginning to feel very uncomfortable.

Two drinks later, the women joined the lads at their table. The game of small talk and banter began. The girls loved the Irish accent, and Neill was putting on one hell of a show for them. John was embarrassed but also getting fairly drunk. The two men stood simultaneously to use the loo and laughed at the timing.

When they were in the toilet, Neill said, "That was perfect timing. I have something to make tonight one for the record books," while reaching into his pocket to retrieve a small foil-wrapped package.

Neill unwrapped the foil to reveal two small blue tablets, shaped like diamonds, on a playing card. John knew these were Viagra because he'd looked into it two years ago when sex was still a thing, but he'd never gotten around to trying it because there was no point these days.

Neill popped one in his mouth, swallowing without water, while handing the other to John. He couldn't believe what was happening. "I'm good; I don't want one," John said, holding his hands up like he was under arrest. He was in total disbelief.

Neill smiled wryly and said, "Wow, I'm impressed you don't need the blue miracle to make yourself last," giving John a playful box on the shoulder as they returned to the table with the two beautiful Spanish women.

John panicked, desperate for a way out of this mess. He played it cool for a while, but he had a plan. A few years ago, he was widely known to suffer crippling migraine headaches. He never told anyone that he was sorted out by spinal adjustments to his neck by a spinologist. He was desperate and willing to try anything. It only took a few months, and he'd never had another headache. He was embarrassed to tell anyone he'd gone to a *quack* and was fixed, so nobody knew about it. This secret was going to be the ace up his sleeve.

John switched to fizzy water for his next drink. Neill looked at him, surprised and asked, "Hey mate, are you okay? The night's still young, and we'll be here a long time."

John rubbed his temples and rolled his head around on his neck. "I feel one of those bloody migraines coming on, no doubt about it. I'm afraid I'll have to say goodnight and head straight to bed, or tomorrow will be a bust," John said while slowly standing and shaking hands with the two women. Neill looked at him in utter disbelief. "Aww, Jaysus, you can't be serious," he said, nodding toward the women.

John shrugged his shoulders apologetically. "It's rotten timing, alright, but I need sleep as soon as possible." He turned towards the door and was gone in seconds, filled with relief.

The women noticed what was happening. After John left, they both closed in on Neill, wrapping an arm around his neck and kissing him on the cheeks. Neill smiled like the proverbial Cheshire cat. Neill was full of himself the following day. He'd spent the night elsewhere and only came into their room to shower, change into golf gear and hit the course. Neill was on a high like John hadn't seen since their 20s. The golf was good, but Neill could only talk about the previous evening with the two beautiful Spanish *birds* at the same time.

"Jaysus John, that little blue pill is one hell of a magic bullet," Neill bragged unabashedly. "We were at it for hours. Let me know if you want details because I'd happily relive last night anytime," he said with a chuckle.

Neill acted like he wasn't married and had no children.

"Nope, not interested mate. Keep it to yourself," John replied. He was flooded with emotions. Envy was top of the list, making him feel *dirty* inside.

The temptation to *have a go,* as Neill phrased it, the next evening was crippling. After all, he hadn't had any meaningful sex beyond the Christmas just past for over a year. John knew nobody would find out. Neill had gone to a local chemist and bought a new box of blue miracles. John knew if he did it, he most likely would never have sex with his wife again because the guilt would eat him up. And with his luck, John was worried he'd catch some disease. John firmly decided he wanted nothing to do with sex on this holiday. Neill believed the fake migraine the previous night, but he must be honest now, so it was clear he wasn't going to *play away.*

"Are you fucking serious? I mean, are you out of yer mind like?" Neill said furiously as he raised his hands in a questioning gesture. "What the hell did you think this holiday was about? Golf? For fucks sake! You bloody better swear not to mention a word of this to anyone, or my marriage is fucked," Neill said, pointing a threatening finger at John.

"You can do whatever you like mate, and I'll say nuttin'. We've been friends far too long to turn into rats. I'm hoping when we return, Helen will have had a change for the better and life will be like it was a year ago," John said matter-of-factly. "Don't be thick! That's never gonna happen. Didn't you notice all the lads in the bar last night? Most of them are here for the same reason I am, and I'm not going to waste an opportunity when I get one," Neill said as he marched past John, slamming the door behind him.

John wished he could ring Helen, if only to hear her voice. However, he didn't want to disturb her retreat, and he didn't know what he would say, so he sat on the bed and waited until it was time to eat. He thought deeply about what life was like in the past and how desperately he yearned for it to return. Following a lonely dinner, John turned in early, looking forward to the golf the next morning.

Neill hadn't slept in his bed the previous night, so John knew Neill had found another *date*. John was both angry and envious at the same time. He longed to feel intimacy again. John went to breakfast and hoped to see Neill because he felt so lonely. His mate wasn't anywhere to be seen, and their tee time was in one hour. He ate breakfast, returned to the room and rang Neill to check if he was already on the putting green or in the pro shop.

Neill answered, sounding like he'd just woken up. "Sorry, John. I should've sent you a text. I'm going to spend the day with the woman I met last night. We get on like a house on fire, and I won't be back tonight. Sorry again," Neill said, hanging up before John had a chance to say anything.

John was gobsmacked. He felt numb, angry, heartache, despair and confused all at the same time. Seething anger and regret for the trip surfaced as he dropped three balls on the putting surface to begin the warm-up for the round he was about to play alone. John was looking forward to this holiday. He was anticipating some good conversations with Neill. He had even bought two new sets of golf clothes especially for the trip. Livid didn't go far enough to cover the emotion John now felt towards Neill.

A gentleman who appeared to be a few years older was doing the same on the other side of the green. The lad occasionally looked at his watch and the clubhouse door as if waiting for his golfing buddy. The door swung open, a lovely, mature woman strolled across the green, and his face lit up. They had a small chat and shared a meaningful kiss. When she turned to walk away, he playfully grabbed her bottom and squeezed it. She jumped and laughed as she floated back inside the clubhouse.

John wondered what the particular story was there. They didn't act like many mature married couples he knew. John assumed she was a golf holiday girlfriend like Neill had found. As he picked up his balls from the green, a ball rolled near him. It was putted by the lad who had just lovingly grabbed the backside of the beautiful woman. The man came over, collected his ball, smiled a very friendly smile, and extended his hand. The man had hit it that far on purpose. They shook hands and introduced themselves to each other. Charles was from England, and this was his first day of holiday and the first time he had golfed on this course.

"Would you mind if I joined you and your mate for the round? I won't hold you up, and I simply hate golfing alone," Charles inquired. "The lad in the pro shop said there were only two of you out next, so I thought I'd chance asking."

"You're more than welcome to join me. I'm solo today as my mate has other, unexpected, plans today," John responded.

They shook hands, wished each other luck and teed off. Both hit their drives to the same general area on the first fairway, so they began *the walk and talk* of golfers on the way to their second shot. "I'm a semi-retired running coach and a nutritionist," Charles replied after John had inquired what he did for a living. That explains his physical appearance, John thought to himself. Charles glided rather than walked. He was curious about the woman on the practise green. "Are you married?" John asked.

The gentleman's eyes lit up. "Happily, you saw her just before we teed off," Charles answered.

The lovely woman, full of playful passion, was his wife. John was very relieved to hear this as he didn't know if he could listen to any more *holiday sexploits* on another round of golf. "You both look very happy together," John said. Charles laughed, "We are now, but it wasn't always that way." John was curious about what he meant, but didn't press the issue until they finished the front nine. Since no groups were behind them, they decided to stop into the bar for a pint and a sambo. They began to get comfortable, and the pint hit the spot to loosen their tongues a wee bit more.
"So, Charles, what's the secret to the happiness I witnessed on the putting green?" John asked.

Charles leaned back in his chair and chuckled. "Drugs," he replied. John was shocked to the core because he was imagining the recreational variety. Charles was still laughing as he clarified, "Hormones, to be precise." John was now confused and curious in equal measure. "What do you mean? If you don't mind me asking?" "Not at all, John. I'm happy to explain. I am a coach, after all. The solution came following a very volatile period several years ago when I went on the hunt for anything to help my wife with the transition through the menopause," Charles said. "As a marathon coach and nutritionist, I've spent decades training and helping women of that age who took up running or wanted a better diet as they went through it."

This simple statement opened a flood of memories of the past year. Was Helen going through the menopause? God, was that the problem? Maybe there was hope for his marriage if it wasn't just missing the children. John needed time to process what he'd just learned. They finished the round and decided to have dinner with Charles's wife at their hotel restaurant later that evening. This suited John fine because he didn't want to take any chance of bumping into Neill. John had had enough of his teenage antics, and the couple's hotel was far nicer, so the food would be much better.

John yearned to talk to Helen, but what the hell would he say? He couldn't come right out and say that he knew what was going on with her mental and physical state of being. She wanted to kill him when John suggested a doctor visit last year. This could only end in disaster if he couldn't figure out how to handle this conversation. He was hopeful that Charles's wife might offer some solutions.

John got dressed in the hotel room that his mate hadn't visited since yesterday and went to the lobby to take a cab for the short distance to the other hotel. He found himself both very excited and nervous at the same time about the conversations that would take place that night. John felt that this was one of those *'right place, right time'* moments, and he wouldn't waste it. Charles explained how his wife had slowly changed during the volatile period he described on the back nine holes of the golf course earlier that day. The changes Charles talked about were eerily similar to what

John's wife was going through. He was genuinely hopeful for the first time in ages and was glad Neill had wandered off with his lady friend.

Charles and his wife had booked a table in a far corner of the stunning restaurant so they could speak freely without anyone hearing the topic of conversation. The couple sat across from each other, chatting away, when they noticed John at the entrance. Charles stood, motioned him over to them, and introduced him to his missus, Kate. They shook hands, and they all sat down. A glass of wine was in front of each of them, and a bottle of wine was on the table that Kate picked up and offered to John. He gladly accepted, as he felt he would need some *liquid courage* to get through this meal and conversation.

Kate was charming and more than eager to share the story of her *journey back to herself*, as she called it.
"My mother took her own life when she was fifty-four years old, and it's taken this long to forgive her," Kate explained. "I understand the feelings that led her to that decision all those years ago," Kate finished.

John felt as if a bolt of lightning had hit him. That very thought had crossed his mind about his wife when he mentioned the doctor's visit last year. John was now scared that he was correct in his feelings and for his wife's well-being. He hadn't spoken to her in three days. Was she okay? He panicked a bit, and then he calmed down. He would have received a phone call if there were any problems.

As the evening wore on and the wine flowed, Kate's path to find her way back made sense. She had a background in biology as a secondary school science teacher, so when she realised her body was changing, Kate hit the books to see what was happening. She discovered very little information was available in the traditional science books, so she went to the library.

Kate told John, "I was initially drawn to *natural remedies* instead of the medical hormonal treatments. They only helped because I felt like I was *doing something* to try to cope. But I had to admit that they were really of very little use for what I was experiencing," Kate confided. John began to get comfortable and let Kate continue with her story.

Kate explained, "For a long time on the natural treatments, I had convinced myself that I was feeling good again, but eventually I had to admit that this path wasn't working, and I'd been fooling myself. I had no joy or desire for pleasure, and life had simply lost its zest."

Charles simply sat there sipping his merlot and nodded occasionally to confirm that what Kate said was how he experienced it. John intently listened as she described her research into HRT (hormone replacement therapy) and her first visit to the doctor to try another path.

Kate explained, "It didn't happen overnight, but I did feel better almost overnight because what I felt was immediately happening inside my body, and I didn't have to convince myself of anything. I felt hopeful for the first time in a long while."

Charles gave Kate a wink and a thumbs-up. He nodded again. "It was a major turning point." John now felt the wellspring of hope begin to gurgle up again for the first time since before Christmas. He couldn't believe his luck at being there while listening to two wise people who had been through the menopausal mill and came out happy. John had no doubt now that it wasn't the empty nest causing his wife's misery; it was the menopause.

The evening ended after a beautiful meal and a few more glasses of Merlot. John had never had a vegetarian meal before but found it delicious and thought it must be better than his diet. The couple stressed the hormones weren't miracles, and other healthy choices can enhance the transition, but John knew Helen would want nothing to do with a meatless diet. He decided to eat less meat when he got home. John was dreading seeing Neill when he returned to the hotel room. Hopefully, Neill was honest about not coming back to their room that night. John couldn't face him with his newfound knowledge.

Thankfully, the hotel room was empty. John was surprised at how empty. Everything Neill had brought along was gone, and there was a note saying he tried to ring to explain, but he couldn't get through to his phone. John took his phone out of his pocket and remembered that he had turned it off before the evening began because he didn't want to take a chance of it ringing during the dinner, and he didn't want anything to do with his mate. John switched it on, and there were three voice messages from Neill. The first said that there was a beautiful woman who would love to meet him. The second message said she would leave if he didn't reply soon. The last one said he was coming to collect his gear and would stay a few days longer. Neill said he was in love again.

Neill was in love again? He'd known this woman for only two days. John was tempted to ring Neill and explain his thoughts but immediately reconsidered because Neill had planned this all along. He'd brought Viagra on a holiday without his wife. John clearly understood that Neill wasn't after love, only sex, and John was again very envious that Neill was having physical contact passionately. John had a moment of *fuck off mate, you're a terrible person* that quickly switched to *I feel your pain brother and if you have been as lonely as I've been, I can sort of understand.* This instant self-conversation shocked him. He had disdain and empathy in a flash. John felt a strong urge to get home to Helen.

The next day, John golfed with Charles again. They chatted about other life topics and agreed to get together as couples if the future worked out for him and Helen. He was now thinking intently about how to open this topic with his wife. After all, she had no idea it wasn't the kids leaving that was the trouble. He was 100% sure she was in the menopause, and now he needed her to acknowledge that so they could begin to take steps forward to find any solutions that might help her. John knew this was going to be a very tricky conversation.

John arrived at Dublin airport and waited at the baggage carousel for his golf clubs. He thought about Neill and no longer felt the emotion of anger; now he was back on the home sod. John felt sorry for him. Neill's future would be filled with angst, lies and turmoil. On the other hand, John was hopeful again for the first time since Christmas. Neill would have to find his own way back home whenever he returned from Spain. John decided to be totally honest with his wife about what had happened. It was the only way he could think of to transition to the subject of meeting Charles and Kate, and ultimately...the menopause.

John texted Helen to tell her when to expect him home. He didn't want to ring because he didn't know what to say and didn't want to say anything wrong that might scupper this golden opportunity to help the woman he loved find her way back to herself like Kate had. The nervous anticipation

John felt now didn't even begin to compare to what he felt the night he met Kate to discover the fact that the menopause had now become a part of life. John had no idea that Helen was already *on her way back* as he pulled into the driveway of their home.

John parked the car, looked out of the windscreen, and saw a Goddess at the door frame of their house dressed in a way he'd never seen. Helen was there, much to his surprise, to meet him. She was radiant in herself and looked like the woman he remembered. She was wearing what looked like robes, and he laughed inside because he wondered where she had bought such an outfit. He loved the look and wondered why. John had a funny feeling he wouldn't have to talk her into a vegetarian lifestyle. He intuitively *knew* something had happened on the retreat with Mary.

John quickly opened his car door, stepped out and walked the short distance to the front door. He paused with three feet separating them as he glanced from her beaming face with her hair pulled back into a loose ponytail, down her robe-clothed body, all the way down to her Birkenstock-encased feet, then back up. For her part, Kate put her right hand on her hip and lifted her left above her head as she performed a pirouette. She gave a giggle when she finished as she met John's glazed gaze.

John closed the distance between them with a single long stride as he opened his arms to hug his Goddess. He wrapped his arms around her and squeezed with his spinning head resting on her shoulder. He inhaled deeply a fragrance he'd never smelled before but instantly loved. He squeezed a little harder, remembering how desperately he wanted to contact her when Neill was *acting the maggot,* and inhaled another deep breath of that intoxicating aroma.

"You're gonna break me in half if you squeeze any harder, love," Kate joked. "And that smell is an incense called Nag Champa, it's my new favourite." "Helen, you look amazing," John gushed. Helen blushed and said, "Thank you." John smiled and released his bear hug, then, at the same time, they both said, "I need to talk to you about something I learned on the holiday." They burst into laughter together as they entered the house.

They both excitedly told their stories, laughing at the fact that they had both learned about the menopause in the same week, in different countries, and in entirely different ways. The following five weeks were a rollercoaster. They were eating super healthy vegetarian meals, and Helen was drinking the strangest stuff he'd ever smelled as well as taking all sorts of herbal supplements. Helen was burning incense, and strange tones were emanating from Alexa, like the constant sound of a gong that never stopped.

There was also love, sex, cuddles and intimacy, like years gone by. They frequently spoke about the holiday that changed the world they now lived in. John broke his promise to Neill and spoke freely about his unacceptable antics. Helen mentioned the *separation* classes Mary had taken. They cuddled, snuggled, and drifted off to sleep, and he felt like he was in heaven.

The sixth week began with Helen not feeling well, and she needed to sleep later, as she had in the past. She didn't ask Alexa for the sounds or light incense. She didn't care what was fixed for meals. Helen also shut down all the sex, cuddles and intimacy. It had been dwindling for a week or more at this point. John saw the pattern. He was crushed once again. He knew Helen was doing everything the retreat suggested. It wasn't working. He felt horrible for her and feared that he would have to once again go back to a platonic relationship at best.

The *funk* had returned. John immediately thought of the conversation with Charles's lovely wife, Kate. What Helen was experiencing seemed very similar to her story. John knew he had to bring up the possibly catastrophic idea of visiting a doctor again, but he felt he had an ace up his sleeve this time. He called and booked her with a doctor in the UK, Kate had suggested. John figured it was a long shot, but knew he had nothing to lose. John felt like he'd lost already.

"Helen," John said hesitantly, "You know I have no idea what you are going through but seeing you so sad and tired is killing me. Please don't be mad at me, but I've made an appointment with a specialist in the UK who helped Kate," John sheepishly finished. He waited, tense, for the backlash to come. It came. Kate looked up at John through tired yet powerful eyes and asked, "How dare you? What gives you any right to make appointments for me for something that only affects me!!!"

John couldn't meet Helen's gaze. He glanced down at his clasped hands, watching his thumbs nervously chase each other in spiralling circles. He quietly cleared his throat and softly said, "Sorry love, it's not only you affected by this. I didn't mean anything bad by it. It just feels like a good omen that I met Charles and Kate where I did, when I did."

Kate's demeanour softened slightly at this. She considered what John said and still wanted to lash out with another inflammatory reply at his action, but unexpectedly, the weight of understanding then fell upon her, like a massive water balloon splashing her suddenly awake. Kate reflected on the recent weeks when she tried to follow everything the retreat advised. She admitted to herself that she needed something else. Her body softened more until her shoulders slouched forward.

Kate shook her head to break the spell of the moment. She straightened her spine, pulled her shoulders back and stretched out her arm to lift John's chin to meet her gaze and said, "Well, let's not waste a good omen, so."

They landed at Heathrow Airport and were met by Kate at the arrivals hall. When they met, John gave her a big hug and introduced Helen. Kate looked into Helen's eyes and smiled a warm, reassuring smile. The two women embraced like old friends, and Kate reassuringly said, "You're going to see the best specialist we could find. Everything will be okay." "Thank you," was all Helen said in reply.

They brought only carry-on cases, so they headed to the car immediately. As they drove the forty-five minutes to the house, Kate and Helen had the standard cordial conversation of two strangers quickly becoming friends. There was no talk about *the elephant in the room.* Kate decided to let the doctor do it. John stayed quiet.

Charles was just finishing a training session with an extremely fit woman who appeared to be in her mid-forties. They later found out this woman was fifty-eight years old and began marathon training when the menopause started at thirty-nine. She had been twenty-two kilos heavier. Her only *treatment* for her transition was simply running like a woman possessed. She passed through the menopause and became a reasonably well-known distance runner in her class in the UK. John looked at Helen and noticed maybe a spark of hope ignited somewhere deep inside.

They put their cases in the spacious spare bedroom, which would be their home for the next while as they embarked on the quest to find the perfect combination of treatments and therapies to help the most. They hadn't booked a return flight. They were prepared to stay as long as necessary. John thought back and just couldn't believe they were on the cusp of possible solutions which came about because his horny friend missed a tee time over two months ago. What a long, strange trip it's been, he thought. John was excited to see what the next few days would bring, nervous that there wasn't anything that could be done to help his Helen. But he squashed that feeling each time it tried to surface.

Their doctor's appointment was two days away, so they relaxed for the rest of the afternoon. The two couples took a walk together that evening before dinner. Charles was leading the conversation. "Diet and fitness are crucial to the success of my clients," he explained before adding, "Most are also on a hormonal programme."

John and Helen understood this because the five weeks spent eating healthy changed their moods and energy levels. They weren't interested in training for a marathon, but both knew they could do much more for their fitness. When Helen had stopped her walks last year, she needed more and more time in bed. The puzzle pieces were fitting together for the two of them now.

Of course, the dinner that evening was vegetarian and delicious. Charles said, "It isn't necessary to be a strict vegetarian, but eating less meat is better for the body."

They got along like long-lost friends. John was so grateful they were doing something, anything, to help Helen. They both had a couple of glasses of wine that evening as the sun hung low, then retired early to wake for a sunrise walk with Kate, as Charles was training a group of runners.

John and Helen cuddled each other to sleep that night for the first time in over two weeks. It felt amazing to him, and he hoped his wife felt the same.

The next day was a relatively low-key affair. John and Helen walked, ate good meals, and took in the local sights. They barely mentioned the appointment the next day, but they both knew that each was thinking of nothing else. They went to bed early and woke for another walk the next morning. Kate and Charles were busy that day, so John booked a taxi to take them to the clinic. They had no idea what to expect, but they were hopeful as the automatic door to the clinic opened. They checked in at the reception desk. John noticed he was the only man in the waiting area. Nearly every seat held a woman who was trying like hell to get their life back, he thought.

The nurse called Helen's name. They both stood and walked towards the nurse, who had a surprised look on her face. She said it's rare for a partner to attend the consultation. John thought about Neill. He'd never consider attending an appointment like this. John was beginning to realise that getting through this stage of life takes the effort of both partners if they want to be as happy as possible going forward.

The doctor appeared to be in her late forties, and Helen was relieved to see that the person treating her was likely going through the menopause as well. Helen relaxed a tiny bit. She was honestly expecting a male. She wouldn't have been able to relax if that were the case. The doctor began the consultation with standard questions about previous health issues, medications, sleep patterns, and other relevant details. Helen was asked about her menstrual history, childbirth and postpartum. The doctor then quizzed her about her younger sister and her mum. Then asked about diet and alcohol intake. The last part of the consultation focused on how exercise helps the mind/body connection through the change.

The consultation was straightforward. Helen was happy that she had taken care of her fitness fairly well for so many years, as obesity and a lack of fitness seemed to be significant negatives during this time. The next phase of the appointment consisted of taking blood samples and stepping on some scales. The kind nurse handed Helen a folder on the various treatments that would be considered based on the blood work results in the coming days. The doctor was honest, stating that it may take a few attempts to see what works best for her. Helen took the folder and booked an appointment for two days later. She and John left to get a cab back to the house.

They both felt slightly overwhelmed, as everything seemed to happen quickly after such a slow build-up. Charles and Kate were due home in a few hours, so they decided to sit in the back garden and review the information in the folder together. Helen took out the first page, titled *"HRT What You Need To Know."* They read it together, surprised at the multitude of options available.

John looked at Helen with raised eyebrows. "I thought HRT was a tablet you take in the morning or sometime during the day like an aspirin," he said. Helen laughed out loud and said, "I was thinking the same thing."

They realised just how little either was prepared for this time of life. Neither knew that HRT is a cocktail of treatments taken at different times of the day or even on other days of the week in various forms. They learned about oestrogen, progesterone, and testosterone, as well as the roles these hormones play in a woman's life cycle.

The more John and Helen read, the more comfortable they became with the different terminology. They were much more prepared for their next visit to the clinic. They checked in and waited for her name to be called. The doctor went over a list of treatments that would possibly suit her. It was decided to begin with a mild dose of oestrogen in a patch and progesterone in tablet form. The doctor said the low dose to start with won't overwhelm her body as it's very low in oestrogen. Helen would return in three months, and they would reassess the situation.

When John and Helen got into the taxi, she laughed out loud. John asked, "What's so funny?"

Helen said, "After everything we've read over the past two days, it actually does boil down to a tablet daily with this little patch."

Helen was in a good mood, and he shared her joy, but John had seen her like this a couple of times in the past year and kept his hope in check. He clearly heard the doctor say this was a place to begin. If it were a magic bullet, there would be no reason for follow-up visits other than an annual set of blood tests, but he was happy, and she was happy, and they enjoyed the mood. The cab dropped them back at the house. They packed their bags for the evening flight back to Dublin.

Kate was returning home as the car pulled up to take them to Heathrow Airport. The two women hugged deeply, saying they'd see each other in three months. Kate leaned close to Helen's ear and said something that immediately changed his wife's expression. As they got into the taxi, she was quiet and looked worried.

"What's wrong?" John asked with concern etched across his

face. Helen said, “Kate said to be patient; it took her over a year to figure out the best HRT for herself. I sort of assumed we were near the finish line, not the starting line.” She spoke. “I now remember Charles called the period Kate saw the doctor *a volatile period.*”

The first week seemed to go reasonably smoothly, except for a slight, dull throbbing headache that began early in the afternoon and lasted until Helen went to sleep. Helen also noticed that she seemed to be feeling bloated, and her belly would be more prominent at night than in the morning, but she did feel like she was sleeping a bit better. The second week wasn’t quite as smooth. Helen remembered when she began her periods as a teenager and how she was crippled with headaches sometimes for days at a time. It was happening again. She would wake up with a throbbing headache, and it would get worse as the day went on. The nausea also began in week two. It wasn’t too bad, but coupled with the headaches, it was too much on some days, and she had to stay in her room.

John began to get concerned as Helen seemed to be going downhill, so he retrieved the information packet they received on the first visit to the clinic. He studied it. The first time he looked at the pages, the information had no real meaning or context. It did now. He read all about the affects her specific prescription might cause initially. Helen was getting many of them. He did relax a little when he read the symptoms, usually calm down when the body gets used to having oestrogen again. It said it could take weeks or months, or sometimes the treatment needs to be altered to help. He was hopeful it would only be weeks for his wife.

The next six weeks were very difficult, but Helen said the headaches had eased, and nausea was no longer a significant problem. She turned a corner around week eight and began having more energy and fewer headaches. She still had no genuine desire for intimacy, and affection was the last thing on her mind while riding the HRT rollercoaster. John did his best to assist in any way. He could see the changes for the better, and he now understood that this process could take several more months to figure out the best course.

The positive thing John could see was that Helen was becoming happier day by day. Helen was grateful her excessive bleeding had stopped, and her skin didn't itch like it used to. She never experienced extreme hot flushes before the treatment, and anything that she did appeared to stop almost entirely at about week seven. Unfortunately, this was all the positives up to this point. John was playing a very lonely waiting game as her body continued to adapt to the treatment. He was anxious and nervous leading up to the return to the London clinic in a few weeks, and he chuckled to himself about how normal all this had become. Four months ago, they literally knew nothing about the menopause, and now he asked his wife about her bleeding patterns. Another internal chuckle.

Exactly three months after their last visit to the clinic, John and Helen were back in the same room, going over his wife's diary from the past twelve weeks. He knew she was keeping one because she'd write in it each evening, but he'd never read it. Sitting in the far corner, watching his wife and the doctor review the dates and entries, it sounded to him like some pretty grim content.

However, when they finally finished, the doctor looked at Helen, smiled, and said this was a good platform for tweaking the dosage and adding another ingredient.

This surprised John. Helen looked over and gave a weak smile, but her eyes looked hopeful. She finally understood that getting the HRT correct for herself was a lengthy process. And John secretly put *hope* on the front burner because he saw a twinkle he hadn't seen in a long while. The appointment ended with only a tiny addition of a gel testosterone. The doctor said his wife's body had adjusted to the hormones again, and now it was time to introduce one last ingredient. Hopefully, this would restore balance. The taxi ride to Heathrow was calmer than any other they'd had since they began this quest. There was a clear direction and a sense of hope ahead. John looked at Helen and gave a small chuckle.

"What's so funny?" Helen asked with wide eyes. "Not so much funny, but more ironic," John answered. "Remember when I told you how much I regretted the golfing holiday when Neill didn't come back to the room on the second night?" "Yeah. You would even get a bit red in the face when you talked about it," Helen responded.

"Well, here's what I find funny. If Neill had come back, we'd have golfed together that morning. You and I wouldn't be in this car right now because I'd have never had that chat with Charles," John finished.

Helen smiled and leaned her head on John's shoulder. "Thank you for going on that trip and for all your patience, good omens, wha?" Helen said as she got comfortable.

The sailboat was coming into the harbour after a day around the coast of the Dublin area. It was a sunny day, and the sea smelled briny; it was perfect. The heat was welcome as it's usually cold in St. George's Strait. The occasional sea spray was welcome on his face. John looked over at his wife of twenty-seven years and saw the same beauty now as he did all those years ago when they were introduced to each other by a mutual couple, Neill and Mary. It's sad, he thought to himself, that their friends are now divorced, and they hardly ever see them any longer. John now knew the marriage fell apart when Mary was going through the menopause. He didn't know that then. Nobody understood what was going on. He'd hardly even heard that word, as nobody ever talked about it. He smiled at Helen, and she smiled back. John counted himself a fortunate man to have such a happy ending.

FOG-OUTS

By Catherine

Cora pulled her car over to the hard shoulder, put it in neutral and pulled the handbrake. She looked around at the countryside and couldn't for the life of her figure out where she was or why she was there. Suddenly, she remembered she was driving to her friend's house for the weekend in Mayo. She took her phone out to see how much farther it was and was shocked to discover that she was heading to Cork instead. She was on the wrong motorway entirely, and she'd been on it for over twenty minutes. She took a few deep breaths and tried to remember even getting to her current spot. She relaxed a little as she recalled a few unique cars and three lorries that were the same about ten minutes ago. But she couldn't imagine how she would have taken the wrong exit and stayed the course so long.

She set the destination in her phone, even though she had been there countless times, and resumed the drive. As she refocused her attention on the correct route, she reflected on the past two years and how many times she'd gotten lost or forgotten why she was in the room she was in. A bit of panic tickled the bottom of her spine because her grandmother had severe Alzheimer's before she passed away and had no grasp of her surroundings for the final year of her life. She tried to picture herself in a situation like that as she passed by a massive Hawthorne tree on the side of the road that a farmer decided to let be its magnificent self. She said out loud that she'd rather crash into that magical tree and die than ever be like her Nanna. As a young girl, Cora never did very well in school, but she had a brilliant memory. Any assignment that required memorisation was assimilated in one read. Any assignment that required thinking or understanding came very hard to her. She wasn't sporty; in fact, she was a chess geek. Her memory allowed her always to be several steps ahead of poor players and at least one or two steps ahead of good ones. Cora rarely lost a match after the age of twenty-five. She was a bookkeeper by profession, but chess was her passion. She knew she was gifted with a memory that was better than that of other people because they just couldn't see the chessboard like she could. She had every move in every situation by every great chess master memorised, and she absolutely annihilated her opponents for many years.

As she drove on the correct motorway, she allowed her mind to wander. Cora recalled shaking hands with her opponent and congratulating him on his victory. She knew she'd lost the match but had only misty memories of anything that happened during play. She had been losing more often in the past year than ever before, but the competition was getting younger and better, thanks to the internet. Cora told herself that she just needed to focus harder, like she used to. She was forty-five and feeling older. She had to get reading glasses last year, and both of her hips were sore all of the time. She knew she should walk more, and the chess tournaments could incorporate relentless hours of sitting. She was a heavy woman, and no matter what or how little she ate, Cora somehow managed to put on weight.

The real wake-up call occurred during one of her chess lectures. Cora taught classes to eager students and had been doing so for fifteen years. The lecture part of the class hadn't really changed over that time, so she could give the introduction speech in her sleep. Halfway through the speech, in mid-sentence, her mind went blank. She stood in the function room of the library in front of seven students with her mouth open to speak, and she couldn't for the life of her remember what she was saying. She made a joke about being on autopilot for so long that she got careless and forgot. That word again. She never forgot anything. But she was doing so now. She called it *fogging out.* Cora was worried about her mental faculties. The fog-outs continued to increase in frequency over the next few months. Something was constantly tickling the back of her mind. It was thoughts of her Nanna and how horrible life was for her as her mind drifted away. She would soon have to see a specialist.

Cora turned the air conditioner on high in the car as she drove. It was winter and freezing outside, but she was boiling up inside. She knew she was overweight, and she assumed that was why she was hot. It was so bad at night that she had two fans blowing, and she rarely used any covers. She put the indicator on, turned into the Tesco car park, and just sat trying to remember what she was there for. She began to cry for the first time over the fog-outs.

Cora left her appointment with the GP as a bag of mixed-up emotions. After taking her history, he asked a few surprising questions. It was as if he knew exactly what she'd been going through. When he said it wasn't Alzheimer's, she was relieved. When he said it was the menopause, she was shocked. She had heard of the menopause, of course, but knew next to nothing about it. As far as she knew, it was what older ladies got. She wasn't even forty-six yet. She was still young in her mind. The GP assured that her age wasn't uncommon at all, and many women begin even earlier and suggested that she change her diet to lose weight and start swimming or cycling to get fitter. The well-informed GP also suggested taking some blood samples to determine the best course of action to assist Cora with hormonal balance which her GP explained could contribute to symptoms like brain fog and gaining weight which was difficult to shift. Cora was grateful to be in the care of a doctor who was well educated on the subject. As she sat in her car decompressing, Cora vowed she was ready to begin swimming as the cooling aspect of the water appealed to her but struggled with the diet aspect.

Cora had been an ethical/spiritual vegetarian for over thirty years, and although she didn't eat a lot of greens, she kept her portions down to what she thought was proper. She wanted her memory back, and the GP suggested a different diet might help. She booked an appointment with an expert. The nutritionist Cora was seeing asked about a typical week of meals, how much liquid intake and what type. The chat about alcohol was interesting. She wasn't a big drinker, but she liked a pint or two of Coors Light in the evening. The nutritionist explained there was nothing light about beer. Spirits were a better choice for an evening tipple. Beer makes you big and Gin makes you thin, she was told, and they laughed out loud. The real shock came when the nutritionist said that her body isn't doing well without meat in her diet. Cora recoiled because she knew there was no way she would ever eat meat. However, when the nutritionist linked fish oils and memory studies, she paid attention. Nutrition doesn't care about moral values, she was told. The body needs what the body needs. Some thrive without meat. She was told that she wasn't such a person.

The salad in front of her didn't look too bad, but it didn't look like roasted potatoes, either Cora thought. It was the plate next to the salad that she was looking at with a hairy eyeball. A medium-sized piece of white fish was waiting there. The fish was sitting in its own oil, accompanied by lemon and butter. She desperately hoped the magic oil might help with the fog-outs. They were frequent enough that she was driven to try this. Cora reasoned that if the fish was already dead, and she didn't kill it, and if no spirit existed in the flesh, there couldn't possibly be karmic implications. The fish ate healthy food to make its flesh, and now she needed its flesh to make her mind and body healthy. Cora couldn't believe she was about to eat meat for the first time in three decades. She was sure she'd throw up or have some kind of reaction. Neither happened and she found the taste pleasant. The one small tablet Cora took every evening helped her get a better night's sleep and the spray she applied to her lower arm diminished the hot flushes. She still had them sometimes, but the hormones were definitely helping. She ate fish every second night for two months and upped her veg and salad intake.

The clothes that were once tight became a perfect fit, then loose, in a short period of time. Her hips hurt less, and she began to incorporate weight training into her swimming routine. She was still playing chess and was feeling good again, and she resumed teaching classes because the fog-outs were becoming less frequent. When they did happen, she would laugh out loud and blame them on the menopause. She was coming back to herself.

Three years on, and she was half her body size. Cora ate fresh fish as a staple and occasionally chicken. She could never imagine eating red meat. Her body felt good, and her hips rarely bothered her. While Cora still enjoyed the meditative aspect of swimming, she lifted weights and did class strengthening sessions in a nearby gym. Thinking back to when she was sitting on the motorway to Cork, on her way to a different destination, she thought about her Nanna once again. What if it wasn't Alzheimer's? What if she, herself, hadn't gotten the treatment and nutritional support? She could've been committed to an institution just like Nanna. This was sobering and saddening. There was something that could have possibly helped, but very few doctors had been educated about the menopause and offered no treatment options. Her granny was offered Valium or Lithium and told it was depression.

Cora's shroud of fog had slowly lifted, and her memory was continually improving enabling her to regain her chess champion crown and say farewell to the fog-outs.

About the Author

Dr. Michael D. Meyer was born and raised in the Midwest of the USA. Michael graduated as a chiropractor from Palmer College in 1994.

He immigrated to Australia for three years to learn, teach and practice spinology. Dr Meyer moved to Ireland in 2006 and has been in private practice in County Wicklow ever since. Michael is married and has three grown children. He is a first-time author.

Acknowledgments

Many people contributed to the creation of this unique project, and I owe its completion to each one of them. First and foremost, my beautiful and patient wife Susie and her twin sister, my project collaborator, Catherine.

Dr. Mary Helen Hensley planted the seed of inspiration in 2023 following a healing session at her clinic in Athlone. She met me where I was and encouraged me to write what was coming from my head. I did. They were good stories, but very rudimentary. They got better with her help and constant encouragement. There would be no book without her.

My daughter Abbygayl was the first person to read a story besides Catherine. Abby was upset that I had the gall to attempt writing about the menopause. I assured her that if she disagreed with the tone of what I was writing, I would scrap the entire project. She loved what she read, so I ploughed on.

ShadowScript Wordsmiths were brilliant start to finish. As a first-time author they had to literally hold my hand by clearly explaining (many times!) the complex process of specific language useage and possible interpretation every step of the way. In particular, gratitude to Niall the senior editor, who provided a critical review of an early draft and all the subsequent structural edits. He then went one step furter to design my book cover.

To the other ShadowScript edit and review team including Conor and Karen who reviewed various drafts and then handed the final book file over to Susan at Book Hub Publishing to publish this book. They are consummate professionals and I'm looking forward to working with them with for my next few books.

To Book Hub Publishing for taking on my debut book for publication status.

Our families' journeys have been ones of healing and self-discovery, and I hope to provide a space for other families to experience a similar outcome.